American Health and Wellness in Archaeology and History

UNIVERSITY PRESS OF FLORIDA

Florida A&M University, Tallahassee
Florida Atlantic University, Boca Raton
Florida Gulf Coast University, Ft. Myers
Florida International University, Miami
Florida State University, Tallahassee
New College of Florida, Sarasota
University of Central Florida, Orlando
University of Florida, Gainesville
University of North Florida, Jacksonville
University of South Florida, Tampa
University of West Florida, Pensacola

American Health and Wellness in Archaeology and History

DALE L. HUTCHINSON

University Press of Florida
Gainesville · Tallahassee · Tampa · Boca Raton
Pensacola · Orlando · Miami · Jacksonville · Ft. Myers · Sarasota

Copyright 2022 by Dale L. Hutchinson
All rights reserved
Published in the United States of America

27 26 25 24 23 22   6 5 4 3 2 1

Library of Congress Cataloging-in-Publication Data
Names: Hutchinson, Dale L., author.
Title: American health and wellness in archaeology and history / Dale L. Hutchinson.
Description: Gainesville : University Press of Florida, 2022. | Includes bibliographical references and index. | Summary: "In this book, Dale Hutchinson traces the history of American health care and wellbeing from the colonial era to the present, drawing on evidence from material culture and historical documents"—Provided by publisher.
Identifiers: LCCN 2021031888 (print) | LCCN 2021031889 (ebook) | ISBN 9780813069142 (hardback) | ISBN 9780813057996 (pdf)
Subjects: LCSH: Medicine—United States—History. | Medical care—United States—History. | Public health—United States—History. | BISAC: SOCIAL SCIENCE / Archaeology | SOCIAL SCIENCE / Anthropology / Cultural & Social
Classification: LCC R151 .H88 2022 (print) | LCC R151 (ebook) | DDC 362.10973—dc23
LC record available at https://lccn.loc.gov/2021031888
LC ebook record available at https://lccn.loc.gov/2021031889

The University Press of Florida is the scholarly publishing agency for the State University System of Florida, comprising Florida A&M University, Florida Atlantic University, Florida Gulf Coast University, Florida International University, Florida State University, New College of Florida, University of Central Florida, University of Florida, University of North Florida, University of South Florida, and University of West Florida.

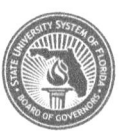

University Press of Florida
2046 NE Waldo Road
Suite 2100
Gainesville, FL 32609
http://upress.ufl.edu

To my father, from whom I learned about the business of pharmacy.
I thank him for suggesting I not practice it myself.
And to my mother, who co-owned and ran Verne's Emporium with him,
And to both of them for teaching me about finance
And the value of labor.

Contents

List of Figures   ix

Introduction: Health and Well-Being in America   1

Part I. American Health and the Colonial Years, 1600–1750

1. Faith, Religion, and Healing in Colonial America   11
2. Domestic Health Care and Informal Specialists   23

Part II. Growing Pains: The Emergence of Specialized Medicine, 1750–1850

3. The Rise of Institutional Care   45
4. Licenses and Liabilities: Medical Training Becomes Formal   65
5. Suspect Specialists   82

Part III. Reformation and Reconstruction, 1850–1900

6. The Civil War and the Reformation of American Medicine   97
7. Ventilation, Germs, and Hygiene: The Post–Civil War Reform   115
8. Hospital Reformation and Redirection   130

Part IV. The Road to Well-Being, 1850–1900

9. Self-Help Meets Regulation: Patent Medicines, Personal Care, and Professional Regulation   149
10. Making Oneself Better: Vitamins, Diet, Exercise, and Other Fads   168

Conclusion: The Road to Wellness   183

Epilogue   187

References Cited   191

Index   209

Figures

1.1. Ceramic bowl with Kongo Cosmogram on base   18
2.1. Distillation by means of a metallic still   25
2.2. Parturition chair   34
2.3. Dentist's key   40
3.1. Urethral syringe recovered from the ship *Queen Anne's Revenge*   49
4.1. Mortsafes at a churchyard in Logierait   70
4.2. Fisk metallic burial case, circa 1850   71
5.1. Scarificators and lancets   84
5.2. Items from Feature One, Dr. Morrogh's Well   93
6.1. Typical pavilion hospital building plan   100
6.2. Satterlee Hospital   102
6.3. Patients at Harewood Hospital in Washington, DC, 1864   102
6.4. Administration of anesthesia   107
6.5. Surgical kit typical of a field physician   108
6.6. Successful amputation of the left hip joint   109
6.7. Embalming fluid bottle   111
6.8. Embalming kit   111
7.1. Design for an earth closet to sit within a commode   127
7.2. Moseley folding bathtub, circa 1880–1900   128
8.1. Tranquilizer chair of Benjamin Rush   136
8.2. Northern Michigan Asylum, Building 50   138
8.3. Northern Michigan Asylum Men's Ward sitting area   138
8.4. Aerial View, Northern Michigan Asylum, Building 50   139
8.5. Men's dining room at the Traverse City State Hospital   141

8.6. Three second-story sleeping porches 143
9.1. Lydia Pinkham's Vegetable Cure advertisement 150
9.2. Hamlin's Wizard Oil advertisement 153
9.3. Pill roller 156
9.4. Stabler-Leadbeater apothecary display 157
9.5. Stabler-Leadbeater office and stockroom 158
10.1. Hydropathy treatment 171
10.2. Deformed ribs due to corset wearing 177
10.3. Exterior view of the Battle Creek Sanitarium 180

Introduction

Health and Well-Being in America

> For everywhere we look, there is work to be done. The state of our economy calls for action: bold and swift. And we will act not only to create new jobs but to lay a new foundation for growth. We will build the roads and bridges, the electric grids and digital lines that feed our commerce and bind us together. We will restore science to its rightful place and wield technology's wonders to raise health care's quality and lower its costs.
>
> (President Barack Obama, First Presidential Inaugural Address, Delivered January 20, 2009)

Health care permeates every aspect of American life, as espoused by then–President Obama. In the post-Obamacare nation, how we provide health care for the masses, and how we engage a range of issues from acute illness to the maintenance of well-being is constantly in the news, debated in the Senate, and subjected to public scrutiny. Advertising for cholesterol-reducing drugs, erectile dysfunction remedies, and fitness centers all serve witness to our commitment to living better and longer, as well as to emptying our pocketbooks. According to the World Health Organization (WHO), health care comprised an average of $9,403 per person in the United States, or 17.8 percent of the gross domestic product (GDP) in 2016.

I witnessed many trends in health care as I grew up and worked in our family pharmacy. We lived above our drugstore and the doctor's office that occupied the other half of our building. From this vantage point, I witnessed a constant flow of patients and customers seeking cures, contraptions, and correctives that made me acutely aware in my adolescent years of the marriage of health care and consumerism. My father was trained and operated his pharmacy at a time when a fair portion of the prescriptions he filled had to be compounded by him. Mortars and pestles, scales, and graduated cylinders were still a part of providing medications, sometimes custom-made, in every pharmacy.

Yet, in our northern Michigan village of 500 people, family cures were perhaps even more numerous and pervasive than those that could be found bottled and dispensed by experts. That curious blend of those who provide health care, those who need it, and practices originating from both the medical profession and traditional home cures have been part and parcel of American health care from the earliest days of the colonies. American medicine, however, did not originate as a package, but rather came into its own after a long period of amalgamation and compounding.

From the earliest colonial intersections of religion and health to the institutionalized and managed health-care facilities of the twentieth century, American medicine embodies three main trends in health and well-being. The first is the mixing and melding of three previously distinct traditions and practices of health care: Native American, African, and European, which after a couple of centuries emerged as American care of health and well-being. The second trend was tied to the radical landscape and built environment transformations that contributed to class differences in health risks, health treatments, and well-being. The third is the emphasis on individual responsibility and personal choice set within a managed health-care system. The latter trend is often reflected in a partnered tension between self-help practitioners and specialists.

How to Use This Product

In this volume, I explore several historical narratives and material correlates that pertain to the growth and development of American health care. Those narratives are neither exhaustive, nor do they strive to achieve textbook cohesion. Rather, they traverse several interlocking topics that pertain to our past and current views on medicine and health. In order to construct those narratives, I employ primary and secondary historical documents, material culture, archaeological data, photographs, and several other sources to present an overview of the development of the American healthcare system.

There are those who would argue that some of those sources of data are better or worse than others. Take historical documents, for instance. Historical documents have long been known to carry substantial bias in their reporting. I would certainly not challenge that contention, nor would I contest the fact that other sources of information, archaeological data, for instance, can often present new insights and interpretations about such things as gender and class differences that are obscured in historical documents.

However, I have previously argued and still contend that no sources of information about the past are unbiased. Archaeological sources are just as biased as historical ones, but in different ways:

> Archaeological remains also suffer from problems of accuracy—usually only a portion of the original materials is preserved, or their remains represent accumulations over long time periods, or the original context has been altered either accidentally or purposefully. No matter what, depictions of the past are probably biased in some fashion. Like the visual art presented through the lens of the artist, historical documents and archaeological remains present only one view of a past situation, one snapshot. The view is not complete, and whether by conscious intent or accidental preservation, only some of the original content and context is present. (Hutchinson 2016: 8–9)

One can only make the most accurate reconstructions of past events and populations by considering the entire suite of archaeological and documentary evidence.

Mapping the Journey

I focus the narrative conversations in the book geographically on the eastern United States and temporally between 1600 and 1950. I do this because they are the geographic and temporal areas I know best in terms of scholarship. As well, there are several books already on health and well-being that focus exclusively on the western United States (for example, Bethard 2004; Steele 2005). The time periods I include represent the earliest colonial encounters through the major advances in medicine of the first half of the twentieth century. A challenge in writing books that traverse centuries is organization; quite simply, the issue becomes whether to organize by topic or by time period. Most topics, especially those fundamentally tied to discussions of growth and change, traverse multiple time periods. Thus, assigning exact dates to trends and patterns is usually not easy.

Archaeologists often employ a method called *seriation*, which is a relative dating technique. In a nutshell, seriation employs trends in popularity of something such as bottles, shoes, art styles, or even fashion to establish chronology. What one generally finds is that as one variation becomes more popular, another fades out. In much the same way, changes in the material culture and theoretical approaches in health care do not have clean temporal boundaries, and the discussions follow a meandering route at times. I have thus generally contextualized trends in American health care and well-being as meandering, popular, culturally bound phenomena that could often be graphed as a seriation plot.

American health care is rooted in the home, family, and tradition. Despite the recognition that specialists and their tools can provide knowledge and care not possible by the commoner, Americans have often expected to have access to cures created by specialists but administered by the consumer. As well, they have always kept in their arsenal of cures those that are traditional and of natural ingredients. Every stage of technological advance often saw resistance, and only sometimes gradual acceptance. The earliest acceptance has generally been by those who could afford a novel cure or practice, while simple, home-based cures and treatments remained within the pocketbook of the less financially fortunate. Thus, slow growth in medical advance has usually occurred alongside traditional methods and materials.

I look in the first part of the book at the initial century and a half of American health care, with concepts and traditions drawn from Indigenous North America, from Africa, and from Europe that coexisted during the early colonial period. The focus on three ancestral populations is not intended to suggest that other settler populations did not influence American health care. For instance, settlers from China or Latin America made significant contributions to American health care, but I chose to limit my discussions to the populations who predominantly contributed to the early colonial period and then follow them through.

In reference to those three ancestral populations, to use an aggregate term to refer to any of them ignores the immense variability that existed between human ethnic groups and populations that are lumped under a broader cultural tradition, label, or term. For instance, "European" ignores the differences between those from Italy and those from Britain. "Native American" or "Indian" ignores the vast variability between Indian tribal groups and nations. However, my intent is only to discuss some broad concepts that are shared in general ways across the constituents of each tradition while illustrating some general differences between the traditions. I also restrict my usage of either "Native American" or "African American" until after roughly 1750 as those populations did not subscribe freely to being Americans, preferring the terms "Indian" and "African" or "of African descent."

From the three separate cultural foundations and traditions of healing, emergent Americans began to borrow, disseminate, and amalgamate a broad array of approaches to health and well-being. Health and well-being in colonial America was fundamentally tied to the environment and environmental change. Landscape alteration was fundamentally tied to labor, and labor was fundamentally tied to social and economic stratification. In the emergent mercantile economy of America lay the mortar and pestle of health and well-being.

The establishment of rice agriculture in Carolina, for instance, created new breeding areas for mosquito vectors through the massive reconfiguration of inland and tidal river lands. Natural landscape transformation was an essential part of the changing landscape of disease. The built environment went beyond agricultural complexes to the homes placed adjacent to them and served as material witness to the early stratification of risks to health and well-being (discussed in much more detail in Hutchinson 2016).

Social change sculpted the way in which new ideas were incorporated into a developing colonial landscape of home health care. By the eighteenth century, plants known to the Indians were found in use by enslaved communities alongside African plants. There was plenty of opportunity for Africans and Native Americans to share their native pharmacopeia through enslavement, marriage, and shared communal refuge from slavery and exploitation.

The second part of the book discusses the emergence of specialized medicine from roughly 1750 to 1850. Although formal medical training was obtained in eighteenth-century Europe, few of those who had that training came to America in the early colonial years. Rather, the earliest forms of medical training in America were often those obtained through exposure and experience in the home and community. Care was provided in the home, and when help was sought, it was through social relationships with individuals trained through experience, not formal education. At most, formal training was limited to apprenticeships.

With apologies, the narrative trends away from the three ancestral traditions in the second part of the book. Social stratification is partly to blame, because some traditional approaches become more obscured as middle- and upper-class changes in health care become more predominant in the historical records. A narrative about differential access to health care is certainly there, but in large part I explored that topic earlier (Hutchinson 2016). In this book, I explore the major trends in the growth of American medicine with somewhat less focus on the variation in health care by ethnicity.

As the range of challenges to health grew, so did those who specialized in health and well-being. The medical profession became more prestigious and lucrative. In cities like New York, specialists ranged from doctors to sanitation officers, the latter serving as a bridge between public, policy, and poverty. Yet, in many localities domestic medicine continued to play a predominant role in caregiving, and people trained by apprenticeship rather than university were still a major part of the healing profession. Whether via a midwife, an itinerant physician, a quack, or a legitimate surgeon, the tool kits that were part and parcel of the trade became a material symbol of the route to well-being.

A correlate of stratification, increased poverty, and a mercantile economy were the "risky trades," those that placed some individuals differentially at risk for impacts on their health and well-being. State hospitals and almshouses were necessary institutions for care and healing of those who could not afford medical care. While they followed an age-old tradition of providing care, they also reflected America's new social and economic stratification.

The tension between medical specialists and those who stressed home health care reached feverish proportions during the first half of the nineteenth century, a time of intense criticism of the American medical system by the Thomsonians and others. The failure of care institutions and an absence of medical knowledge all converged to create a health-care crisis about 1850.

The third part of the book explores the reformation of American care of health and well-being. Almost as if a response to the health-care crisis, the Civil War (1861–1865) brought about reformation out of necessity in order to accommodate the immense number of sick and wounded. The four-year period of the war was one of reform in medical treatment, hygiene, and surgery. The changes brought about by the Civil War inaugurated a new intensity about the many ways one could make improvements in health.

Hospitals and hygiene were two major areas of reform. Fundamental issues such as clean water, air quality, and disposal of biological wastes became major reformation movements in the eighteenth and nineteenth centuries in America. As well, specialized hospitals and care facilities for tuberculosis and mental health care were built upon the changes inaugurated in the late nineteenth century.

Part IV looks at the increased emphasis of self-help health care and the tensions between specialist and nonspecialist. At the same time as major reforms for institutional health care were taking place, health care became all the more visible through the packaging of tonics, pills, salves, and the like. They marked the American trend toward consumerism and self-help so apparent after the mid-nineteenth century. Shortly after 1900, Coca-Cola began advertising their "make you feel better" beverage. Other individuals and manufacturers promoted numerous cures targeted at children to quell crying, vomiting, and restless urges in an effort to procure "restful naps." Many of these packaged curatives circumvented medical specialists and allowed consumer households to directly practice domestic health. The movement was not taken lightly, and those vested in medical specialization met it with strong criticism, the formation of professional organizations, and legal challenges.

Several health fads emphasized diet, exercise, vitamin supplements, and a variety of specialized treatments that could mitigate health insults from anxiety to aneurisms. Aside from home health treatments and membership in clubs, specialized spas and resorts for the well-to-do were popular. That trend is personified by Dr. John Harvey Kellogg who ran a health spa and resort in Battle Creek, Michigan, and whose breakfast cereal figured religiously into a healthy diet. It later became the founding product of his brother's breakfast empire. The trend in self-care was counterbalanced by specialists in health care, and by the facilities where they trained and performed small miracles of treatment and recovery.

A final concluding chapter discusses the changes in American perceptions and approaches between 1600 and 1950. The road to wellness was a long one, and not without growing pains, setbacks, and compromises. Through it all we have tried to balance care provided by professionals with self-administered cures.

* * *

At the crossroads of two distinct approaches to health and wellness, we can do well to look back on the past, which in no small way dictates how we arrived at the present. At one pole is the managed, provisioned, and promised care provided by specialists and specialized health-care facilities. At the other pole is personal practice. At no time in the past have Americans had more access to health-care knowledge. Access to digital archives and personal fitness coaches means that we can do all we can on our own to improve our health and maintain fabulous wellness. On the other hand, there are situations, cancer for instance, where specialists are necessary components of the care process. In the following chapters, we will explore the details of the American tradition of health and well-being as seen through the lenses of historical narrative and material culture.

I

American Health and the Colonial Years, 1600–1750

1

Faith, Religion, and Healing in Colonial America

> The Indians of these Parts use Sweating very much. If any Pain seize the Limbs, or Body, immediately they take Reeds, or small Wands, and bend them Umbrella-Fashion, covering them with Skins and Matchcoats: They have a large Fire not far-off, wherein they heat Stones, or (where they are wanting) Bark, putting it into this Stove, which casts an extraordinary Heat: There is a Pot of Water in the *Bagnio* [sweating house], in which is put a Bunch of an Herb, bearing a Silver Tassel, not much unlike the *Aurea Virga*.
>
> (Lawson 1967: 48)

There has long been a notion that the land that would become America was relatively disease-free before European colonization, and that new diseases introduced from Europe and Africa resulted in the near-extinction of the Indigenous inhabitants. However, as alluded to by Lawson, Europeans noted a rather extensive pharmacoepia and many physical treatment protocols for disease among the Indians. The Indians clearly knew about illness, health, and well-being.

In fact, the Indigenous inhabitants experienced several health impacts prior to colonization, including infectious diseases such as Chagas disease, treponemal infections (bacterial skin infections such as syphilis), and mycotic (fungal respiratory) diseases. New infectious diseases did cause large-scale native mortality, but those new diseases and subsequent depopulation occurred within the context of cultural upheaval during the colonial period and over a 350-year period (see Hutchinson 2016 for much more detailed discussion).

It is probably better to think of the early colonial period as one where people from different places had their own distinct diseases and other health issues, and their own traditional ways and means for dealing with them. Treatments commonly included plant and other chemical compounds, devices for administering treatments and physically altering patient conditions, and consulting informal specialists. The details varied between traditions, but they generally shared all of the above traits. They also each had specific beliefs about the causes of insults to health and well-being, and in each tradition religion played some role.

Indian Approaches to Health and Well-Being

Faith and Healing

It is important to recognize the cyclical nature of the universe perceived by many Indigenous populations of the land later known as America. The world was a continual set of processes that repeated themselves and formed the seasons of being. Divisions between well-being, magic, medicine, spirituality, and ritual did not exist—they were all fundamentally linked together. Reciprocity between humans and humans, humans and the natural world, and humans and spirits were seen by many Indian groups as important factors in maintaining health and well-being. When relationships were disturbed, or actions by an individual or group resulted in disharmony with any of those relationships, disease could be one outcome.

Healers were often those people who facilitated access between the physical, metaphysical, and spiritual aspects of wellness, and who could isolate the causes of disease and the methods needed for healing. The healers were usually medicine men or shamans whose spirituality and powers came from their relationship with the spirits. It was the job of the shaman to determine which spirit was causing the trouble as different curative agents were required for each one (Tedlock and Tedlock 1975; Vogel 1970). They acted as mediators between the individual, the community, and with the spirits and deities.

What Causes Disease?

Indians emphasized that people were generally healthy, but that forces from nature, climate, magic, and spirits could impact health. They believed that bodily function was not purely a physical phenomenon and that spiritual elements played a vital role in shaping health and disease. The Cherokees and the Iroquois, for instance, attributed the causes of several diseases to spirits, although one might refer to them more as syndromes or symptoms, since it was not clear what specific diseases are referenced.

Some nations, such as those inhabiting the Northeast, emphasized the importance of dreams in both causing disease and revealing its causes. Soul loss could occur when the soul left the body during a dream. Father Jean de Brébeuf noted that for the Huron "The dream is the oracle that all these poor Peoples consult and listen to, the Prophet which predicts to them the future events, the Cassandra which warns them of misfortunes that threaten them, the usual Physician in their sicknesses, the Esculpius and Galen of the whole Country" (Brébeuf 1636).

Treating Disease

Indians had lived in the land that would become America the longest, and thus they had the most intimate knowledge of the climate, animals, and plants. Time and time again, Indian knowledge would aid people from other ancestral populations in meeting the same challenges to health and well-being. Indians emphasized physical actions in the treatment of disease. Phenomenological approaches (approaches that concentrate on consciousness and the objects of direct experience, or phenomena) to well-being were therefore emphasized and practiced. Phenomenological approaches included dances; chants; music through singing, instruments, rattles, and drums; incantations; and amulets. Sucking of the ailing parts of the body was sometimes employed in order to remove objects such as animal claws or feathers that were the cause of the ailment. Medicine bundles or bags contained medicinal plants for consumption, as well as other objects used for healng; at times they also channeled "power" to healers. The bags were usually made of cured animal skins, often of totemic animals, and were frequently decorated with symbolic ornaments.

Immersion in smoke, water, or steam, and the act of sweating in a closed structure, were important cleansing and healing activities. The Powhatan, a confederacy of tribes impacted by European colonization, and many other groups used sweating as a means of healing. As Lawson (1967 [1709]) mentions, these treatments also were among the methods used to relieve pain. In addition to sweat baths, warm poultices, massage, and aromatic fumigation were among those treatments that relieved pain (Vogel 1970). There is substantial archaeological evidence to support historical accounts of Indian sweat lodges.

Mehta (2007) examined variability and similarity in sweat house architecture, taking "the position that the sweat lodges of the southeastern Indians are a meaningful architectural construct fully embedded within Indian cosmology and religion" (Mehta 2007: abstract). He examined the described features of 29 sweat lodges that were documented historically:

"shape, multi-use or single-use, diameter (span), cultural group, number of people accommodated in the structure, location, proximity to water, depression in ground, orientation of door, construction materials, number of poles, location of the fire, method of heating the lodge, the number of stones (if used), and any medicinal herbs utilized" (Mehta 2007: 30).

From those descriptions, he devised a type-variety model (an architectural grammar; see Mehta 2007 for a detailed description of that model) that elicits a system of rules using types and varieties to account for the multiplicity of sweat lodge forms, and applied that system to features at two North American archaeological sites, Smiley Rock (22AD1041) and Poplar Cove (22AD1040), both in Mississippi. He concluded that the features at both sites were multipurpose facilities which include uses as sweat lodges.

Parks (2018) reported that among the multiplicity of forms documented archaeologically, numerous semisubterranean sweat lodges (SSLs) were found in Ontario and places adjacent to Ontario. She describes the characteristics of SSLs as:

> flat-bottomed pits with a keyhole shape and which contain a ramped entrance leading down into the structure. A basal layer is commonly noted at the bottom of the pit, believed to have been deposited during the use of the structure. The superstructure of the SSL was supported by posts, which are seen in the archaeological record either at the bottom of the pit below the basal layer, or as a ring around the perimeter of the feature. Coverings could have included skins, bark, or sod. At the end of the feature's use, it was filled in with layers of sterile subsoil, sometimes containing lenses of artifact-rich soil. In many instances, surficial refuse layers are noted as very dark brown to black, artifact-rich deposits. It is likely these upper refuse layers were deposited over time, after the SSL was filled, rather than being a rapid infilling event.

Parks was interested in the "life-history" of sweat lodges at the Redeemer site (AhDx-114), a fourteenth-century Iroquoian village in Hamilton, Ontario. Using a series of spatial analyses, she found that "sweat bathing was an important part of the Redeemer community's collective experience, seen in the frequency of SSLs at the site, the standardization of construction methods, and in the deposition of artifacts of significance, together signifying a strong community of practice" (Parks 2018: i).

Indians also knew how to treat fractures through the use of splints and to stop bleeding by using bird down or moss. It was from Indians that Samuel Fuller and three barber-surgeons who arrived on the *Mayflower* in 1620 learned the art of stabilizing fractures with wood or wet pieces of leather to form a splint (Wigglesworth 1980). Discussions of the use of splints include references to the Creek, Iroquois, Ojibwa, Pima, and Apache, to mention a few (Vogel 1970: 50, 215, 352). There are also reports of the use of flint blades for making incisions, syringes of hollow bone used for injecting compounds into wounds, and animal bladders for enemas (Hallowell 1935; Toledo-Pereyra 2006: 6; Vogel 1970: 11).

Internal balance was part of Indian health, and Indigenous populations had long-term knowledge of which plants could be used for specific conditions. More than 200 species of plants in the U.S. Pharmacopoeia are known to have been used for specific purposes by Indian nations (Toledo-Pereyra 2006: 7). Astringents reduce swelling and cause body tissue contraction, and are typically used for bleeding, reduction of diarrhea, or shrinking hemorrhoids. Tannins are natural astringents, and large amounts of tannins are found in hemlock (*Conium maculatum*), wild geranium (*Geranium maculatum*), bayberries (*Myrica* sp.), and oak (*Quercus* sp., especially bark).

Cathartics are laxatives, and some Indian medical lore held that spirits could be evacuated from the body by purging it. Mayapple (*Podophyllum peltatum*) was used by the Cherokee as a cathartic. Most often the mayapple fruit was used, but the root was also employed. Cathartics were often used in conjunction with vermifuges, drugs which kill or expel intestinal parasites. Common vermifuges native to America were Indian Pink (pinkroot, *Spigelia marilandica*), the roots of wild plum (*Prunus americana*), wild cherry (*Prunus avium*), and the seed of Jerusalem oak (wormseed, *Chenopodium ambrosioides*).

Emetics are drugs that induce vomiting, and they were widely used by Indians. The Iroquois, among other groups, used green hellebore (also called white hellebore, *Veratrum viride*) as an emetic. The Virginia Powhatans used various infusions from roots, tree bark, and herbs to purge the body either through defecation or vomiting (Savitt 1990: 9). Other purgatives and emetics included Yaupon (*Ilex vomitoria*) which was consumed as a tea in vast quantities to cause vomiting by Indians in the Southeast (Lawson 1967). Lobelia (*Lobelia inflata*) was known as Indian tobacco or puke weed. When steeped in water, it acted as a purgative.

Lobelia could also be smoked and caused the bronchial tubes to dilate; it was thus used for asthma, whooping cough, and bronchitis (Toledo-Pereyra 2006: 7). Another plant employed for pulmonary ailments by Indians in Virginia was Seneca Snakeroot (*Polygala senega*); it was also used for snake bites. Fever can be reduced by drugs known as febrifuges. Common ones were a wildflower, Boneset (*Eupatorium perperfoliatum*), Joe Pye weed (*Eutrochium purpureum*), and dogwood bark (*Cornus florida*). After it entered trade networks from South America, cinchona (*Chinchona* sp.) bark was very commonly used for fevers.

John Josselyn (1860) wrote extensively about the medicinal cures of New England Indians. Wounds and bruises, he reported, were treated with green hellebore in combination with raccoon (*Procyon lotor*) or "wildcat" grease. Sassafras (*Sassafras albidum*) was also used to treat bruises as was acorn oil, the latter also used for toothache. Indian pinkroot was used by the Cherokees as a vermifuge to treat intestinal worms. Botanical treatments for pain were also used by Indians.

One of the best-known examples is the white willow tree (*Salix alba*), which when ingested was converted to a similar compound to aspirin (acetylsalicylic acid) by groups such as the Ojibwa and Iroquois (Vogel 1970: 393). Mayapple root (*Podophyllum peltatum*) was used by Indians in the Northeast to cure venereal warts (Toledo-Pereyra 2006: 7; Vogel 1970). Dietary deficiencies were often corrected through botanical supplements. It was from Indian healers, for instance, that Europeans learned of spruce (*Picea* sp.) consumption as a cure for vitamin C deficiency (scurvy), and of bearberry (*Arctostaphylus uva ursi*) for the same affliction (Vogel 1970: 42).

Not all botanical drugs were so specialized in their use. Goldenseal (*Hydrastis canadensis*), for instance, was used for sore eyes, sore mouth, and thrush. Tobacco (*Nicotiana* sp.) and sassafras were both aromatic plants which were used by the Southeastern Algonkians in Virginia for the cure of many diseases (Hariot 1972). Both plants became a major component of the early Virginia colonial economy.

African Approaches to Health and Well-Being

Faith and Healing

It seems clear from both historical and archaeological evidence that enslaved Africans straddled Christianity and religious traditions from their homeland. Many, if not most, were originally from the western rim of Africa from Senegal to Angola. While numerous spiritual chants invoked Jesus, enslaved Africans also recognized healers who almost universally attained their healing powers as "gifts" that were connected with divine intervention (Fett 2002: 36; Schwartz 2006). Conjuring was often a part of the healing art, and illness was frequently seen as a rupture in collective relationships of the living and the dead. Thus, both native and African populations saw illness and health as primarily derived from spiritual origins. Health was due to complex relationships that included living people, their deceased relatives, and the "spirit world." Healers were skilled to wield special powers that allowed them to communicate across those relationships.

What Causes Disease?

Disease was often attributed to spiritual causes in African traditions (Fett 2002). Balance of human relationships, and those with the natural and spiritual worlds, were important in health and well-being. In the same way that doctors cited medical training to legitimize their practice, African healers cited spiritual insight, for instance, or being born to be a midwife, or lessons from relatives, usually a mother. Healers frequently emphasized their strong spiritual connection, which contributed to their effectiveness as medical practitioners.

Harmony, however, was difficult to attain given the fact that many individuals of African descent were forced to straddle their own cultural and medical traditions with those of Europeans who enslaved them. Their enslavement ensured that their beliefs about health and the practices for curing disease would remain in many ways less well-documented—most slaves were illiterate and therefore the records about their lives are presented through the eyes of European writers. It is not that there is a dearth of historical narratives, but rather that they are filtered through European interpretations.

Treating Disease

Elder enslaved women of African descent played an essential part of healing in the South. "While age devalued a slave in the market-place and the fields, it provided a significant foundation of authority for black healers within slave communities. The elderly, though a small proportion of the southern enslaved population, were honored for their learning and the services they continued to provide to slave communities" (Fett 2002: 55). Most midwives in the South were frequently elder women of African descent who took care not only of their families but of the extended collective enslaved household. Slaveholding women were frequently involved in the care of ill slaves, generally through visitation to their quarters or the sick house, where they provided medicines and simple physical treatments like lancing boils (Fett 2002: 115; Kemble 1984 [1863]). Plant recipes for healing

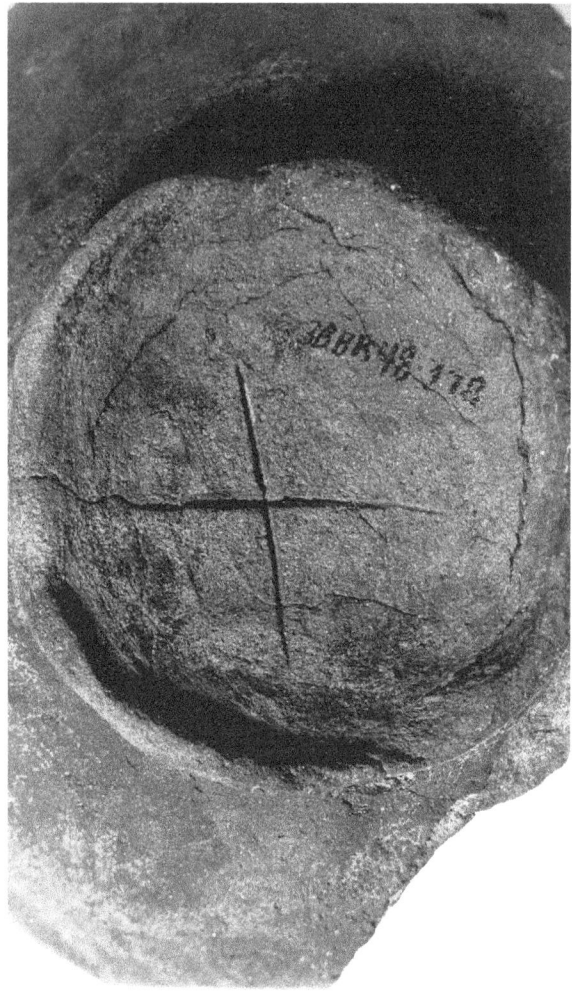

Figure 1.1. Ceramic bowl with Kongo Cosmogram on base. Photograph taken by Emily Short; originally published as Fig. 76 in *Uncommon Ground: Archaeology and Early African America, 1650–1800*, by Leland Ferguson (Smithsonian Institution Press, 1992). I thank Leland Ferguson for permission to use the image.

were frequently drawn from the knowledge of elder African women (Fett 2002).

Most of those recipes came from various plants, as slave medicine was deeply rooted in herbalism. The plants came from both African and Indian traditions and tended to be either locally grown or foraged in the nearby forests adjacent to the fields. Elders born into slavery recalled during interviews voluminous lists of plants that grew locally where they lived. The plants were then used to make teas, ointments, salves, and poultices. Their preparation was deeply rooted in spirituality.

One testament to the connection between herbal cures and spirituality is demonstrated through Colonoware bowls found at archaeological sites along the Cooper River in South Carolina. Colonoware is a broad term that refers to unglazed earthenware manufactured and used between 1750 and 1825 by the people living in the Cooper River region (Ferguson and Goldberg 2019). Thousands of Colonoware sherds have been found at or near the sites of African American habitations.

In 1991, archaeologist Leland Ferguson went to Sierra Leone in the hopes of expanding the interpretations of Colonoware. He showed photographs of some of the ceramics to college students there, proposing that they were food containers. To his surprise, the students responded that they looked much more like the ceramics used to prepare and administer traditional herbal medicines. Through further documentary research, Ferguson discovered that the incised marks on the ceramics are the Kongo cosmogram, often two perpendicular lines, crossing in the middle and within a circle (Figure 1.1; Ferguson 1992, 1999; Ferguson and Goldberg 2019; Fett 2002: 80). The marks indicate a connection to Central African (Bakongo) ritual and, Ferguson argues, clearly indicate the bowls were used ritually for medicine.

Herbs and other plants were not only consumed or ingested. There are numerous accounts of wearing asafetida (asafoetida, also known as devil's dung due to the smell, *Ferula* sp., or nutmeg around the neck to prevent illness and ensure good health (Covey 2007: 74). Garlic was also worn around the neck to promote health, and potatoes were carried in the pocket for the same reason. Plants were also placed in strategic locations of the home; saw palmetto (*Serenoa repens*), for instance, was placed over doorways to remove hexes or curses. Nonplant-based materia medica was extensive and included ants (teething), ash and soot (topical), axes (fending off spirits), coins (fending off numerous ills), charms (conjure), frogs and toads (numerous cures), and many other cures and preventatives.

European Approaches to Health and Well-Being

Faith and Healing

A fundamental difference between Indian and European concepts of the universe was the cyclical nature that Indians perceived, a universe where the participants acted within the universe. Europeans, as participants in western civilization, were much more inclined to see themselves as outsiders acting on the universe. Spirituality was also part of the concept of health and disease among those of European descent. Christianity often is said to emphasize illness as a punishment from God for sins, frequently of individual actors. Violation of religious laws, for instance, was part of the European view of disease, although its importance varied among various regions and religious sects. Unlike those of Indigenous or African descent, however, Europeans looked primarily to the body as a cause of disease, and only when natural treatments did not work did they look further to spiritual causes. Europeans, in fact, cited several different causes of disease, and sometimes beyond individual actors. For instance, collective guilt of a community could result in the wrath of God in the form of illness, and sometimes epidemics were attributed to community sins.

Causes of Ill Health and Well-Being

For the most part, European notions of health and well-being were fundamentally physical. Europeans shared the notion of balance with Indians, but it was rather a balance of internal forces. Those internal forces consisted of four humours—blood, phlegm, black bile, and yellow bile—that were first denoted by the Greek physician Hippocrates. The Roman physician, Galen, elaborated upon them. The humours had various degrees of heat and moisture, and were associated with four elements of the universe: fire (yellow bile), water (phlegm), air (blood), and earth (black bile). Dominant humours varied between individuals and originated from a combination of factors. In general, however, men were hotter than women, and younger people were warmer and moister than those of old age. Many things could upset humoural balance, such as exposure to climate, emotional upset, certain foods, and air quality.

For over two thousand years documents from Greek Hippocratic physicians laid the basis for Western medicine. Both Hippocrates and Galen elaborated on the humoural theory of disease by invoking the role of gases as the carriers of contagion. One of the most influential of those written works was Hippocrates' *Airs, Waters, and Places* (4th or 5th century BCE), which emphasized the importance of environment in disease. As late as the terminal nineteenth century, the standard explanation for disease causation was gases known as "miasmas." So entrenched was miasmatic theory that it was only in the second half of the nineteenth century that it was gradually displaced by the germ theory of disease.

European explanations of disease, however, also included magic and witchcraft. It was the clergy's role to recognize and treat conditions that indicated something beyond natural causes or those from God. Epilepsy, for one, seemed to be one of several diabolical distempers caused by supernatural forces through witchcraft. There were numerous cases in colonial America where witchcraft was assigned as a cause of disease, especially in New England. In Hartford, Connecticut, eight-year-old Elizabeth Kelly was ill and shared some soup with a neighbor woman in 1661. Her health worsened, and she proclaimed that the woman with whom she shared the soup, Goodwife Ayres, was choking her without being present (Tannenbaum 2002: 55–60). The most famous example of witchcraft trials was the Salem witch trials of 1692, when children accused numerous women of causing them harm through witchcraft. European notions of illness, while deeply rooted in the physical, nonetheless also incorporated the role of the supernatural as a cause.

The standard reference guide to diagnosing witchcraft was *Malleus Maleficarum* (Institoris 1486), a text written by two Dominican friars that emphasized both physical and mental damage could be caused by witchcraft. One could suspect witchcraft, according to the text, when the symptoms of disease don't follow normal patterns or when normal remedies are insufficient to resolve them (Watson 1991: 24).

Treating Disease

Prior to 1850, the route to well-being during infectious diseases and other ailments was often focused on emptying the stomach by the use of an emetic that caused vomiting. That process would drive out humours and then a diagnosis would be made regarding what type of humoural imbalance was present. Bloodletting (drawing of blood) was another frequent route to restoring humoural balance. Sweating was often another step to drive out bad humours. Bed rest was essential, and if the early treatments did not ward off a disease, watchers would attend to the patient day and night, making sure that the fires were kept up to maintain sweating and providing "easy foods" such as broth and poached eggs.

Ministers, both through their trust and engagement within the community and their mediation with God, often acted as the healers in colonial America. They would discern the physical signs of illness and diagnose the appropriate mechanism of healing, often through fasting, prayer, and repentance. European healers, whether they were physicians, midwives, or traditional healers, were charged with elucidating the signs of a disease—hot or cold, wet or dry. They often looked to bodily fluids for diagnosis and cures, and they sought to bring about humoural balance through bleeding, purging, vomiting, and sweating. Those approaches were used until the mid-1800s (Toledo-Pereyra 2006: 21).

* * *

Spirituality was linked to health and well-being in the minds of most early colonial people. Spirits, in whatever form one conceived of them, were frequently viewed both as forces causing illness and as revelatory about the cause. At times spiritual forces reached into direct stimulation (control) through magic and witchcraft. It is therefore not surprising that many of the sixteenth- and seventeenth-century healers were also those who attended to the spiritual needs of the community.

European concepts of illness and health, while not divorced from spirituality, focused heavily on physical causes and treatments. Their four humours, and the importance of balance in those humours, aligned with other traditions in the sense that restoring balance was a key to good health and well-being.

2

Domestic Health Care and Informal Specialists

> I cannot deny the honour due to able Physicians and Clergyians when occasion is: Yet we find even that amongst the *Indians,* and all barbarous people, where there is no Men of Learning, the Women are sufficient to perform this duty: And even in our own Nation, that we need go no farther, the poor Country people when there are none but Women to assist (unless it be those that are Exceedingly Poor, and then they have more need of meat than Midwives) the Women are as fruitful, and as safe and well delivered, if not much more fruitful and better commonly in Childbed than the greatest Ladies of the Land.
>
> (Jane Sharp, 1725: xi)

Health care is like an onion; it has several layers that contribute to the whole. At the center is the home, with health care largely administered by women who were, as Jane Sharp indicates, perfectly capable of many health care tasks in the home. Yet, in all three ancestral traditions another layer is occupied by lay specialists who possessed knowledge and skills that made their services desired. Specialists in the care of health and well-being have a long tradition; however, the term "specialist" spans a fair amount of latitude.

For the purposes of this chapter, specialists are defined as those healers whose roles went beyond their own domestic sphere, but who lacked formal, institutionalized training. For instance, individuals who practiced healing within the family are not defined as specialists unless they also made their skills available outside of the household. Specialists could be lay practitioners, such as midwives and doctoresses; or those who had dual roles as healers alongside some other profession, such as clerics. To involve a specialist meant that a household went beyond consulting a published source to actual participation of someone with specialist skills and training.

Domestic Health Care

Women provided the principal means of ensuring household health and well-being in the early colonies. Healing in the sixteenth and seventeenth centuries was an activity that was learned by children from elders. Specialists might sometimes be available, but it was better if women gained experience in caregiving to others. Women were the focal point of household well-being, and they ensured everything regarding health, from hygiene to nutrition; they were essentially responsible for the health and well-being of anyone in the household, including family, servants, and guests.

The above description, however, presents a very Eurocentric picture. The role a woman played in the home varied depending on ethnicity. For those of African and Indian descent, women were often attending to work outside of the home, and child rearing was instead directed by grandmothers and other elders. Nonetheless, regardless of ethnicity, there were many similarities with regard to the nutritional and physical needs of the family.

Care of the Infirm

Health care was often a female communal activity with kin and neighbors participating. Children were frequently immersed in most aspects of domestic tasks that included attending to the ill and ailing. During the seventeenth century and beyond, herbs and other plants were frequently a basis of the healing art. Knowing what medicines to use for what ailments was an essential part of household medicine, as was the provisioning of medicines and food to the ill patient. Much of this information was handed down by word of mouth, although a few multigenerational Euro-American family "recipe books" have been reported (Tannenbaum 2002: 23–26). Family recipes for various salves, ointments, tonics, and other treatments were often handed down through families and friends, and supplemented by the personal and published advice of learned physicians.

Knowledge of the medicinal properties of plants was shared among the differing colonial groups, and names like "Indian tobacco," "Indian Pink," and "Surinam Poison" would often betray the attributed origin of the plant and how to use it. Licorice (*Glycyrrhiza glabra*), a root from West Africa, was used for coughs and fevers, and okra (*Abelmoschus esculentus*) was used for poultices. Jamaican senna *(Cassia obovata)* was used as a laxative, and from America, Jerusalem oak (*Chenopodium ambrosioides*) and capsicum (*Capsicum* sp.) were used medicinally (Fett 2002: 63).

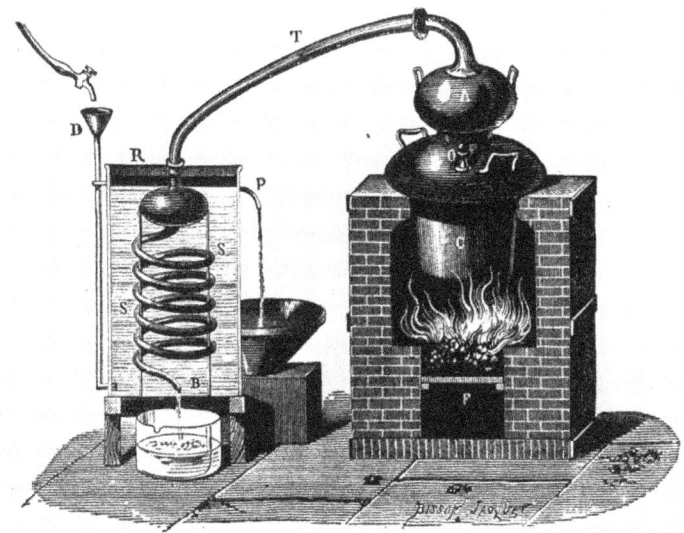

FIG. 4.—Distillation by means of a metallic still. The liquid in C is heated by the fire F. The vapours rise through the head A and pass by the tube T to the worm S placed in a vessel R, through which a current of cold water flows by means of the tubes D and P.

Figure 2.1. Distillation by means of a metallic still. Wood engraving, National Library of Medicine Unique ID: 101435336 (see catalog record), NLM Image ID: A012211.

Many of the medicinal plants were grown in kitchen gardens among vegetables such as carrots and peas which generated the sometimes-used synonym for domestic healing: "kitchen medicine" (Risse 1977; Risse et al. 1977). The preparation of medicines shared many things with the preparation of foods, and again the link to women and kitchens was well deserved. The plants represent a cornucopia of traditional recipes, some used both for food and for medicine.

Medicinal plants were preserved in a number of ways. Drying was one method, and drying in the shade was preferred as the volatile oils, the important part of the plant for medicine, preserved better with slow drying. In other cases, plant essences were extracted by boiling them and condensing the steam, a process known as "stilling," or by infusing them in water, wine, or beer, a process often done in the sun in order to release volatile oils (Figure 2.1). These medicines were then often stored in earthenware pots known as *gallipots* (also called galley pots; Tannenbaum 2002: 27). Other medicines were made to order and included enemas, poultices, teas, and salves which utilized fresh ingredients.

An essential part of caregiving was sitting at the bedside in order to provide for the invalid, to pray if necessary, and to watch for turns for the better or worse. Numerous people were often involved in watching, such as the woman of the house, neighbor women, men, and adolescent children. Medicines were prepared that were appropriate to the disease and they were administered by watchers. The exception to a large cast of watchers was when children were ill. In the case of ill children, the mother was almost always the central watcher.

Care of Children's Health

The health and well-being of children formed an especially important part of household care. Child care began with pregnancy, and for African and European families, was often overseen by a midwife. Consultation with a midwife ideally began after a woman thought she might be pregnant. The midwife would keep in contact with her patient throughout the pregnancy, administering teas, broths, and other treatments that were prepared and provided to ease the pains associated with pregnancy and to maintain a healthy nutritive state. Other treatments were administered to prevent miscarriage, such as black haw root tea (Logan 1989).

After the birth of the child, the midwife would often stay anywhere from a few days to a few weeks with the mother in order to see to her postpartum health, as well as that of the child. In addition to the assistance provided by several other women in the birthing, female children would bathe the child and attend to it while the midwife assisted with the afterbirth and the mother's comfort. Expelling the afterbirth was taken very seriously, and was accomplished in a variety of ways, from having the mother drink buttermilk to blowing into a blue bottle; blue was connected to spiritual practices (Wilkie 2003: 135–137). Postpartum cleansing was often performed by using a douche. Educating the new mother involved first establishing breast feeding, and then incorporated cleaning the child, the correct ways to handle it, and the basic skills of mothering a young baby.

Breast feeding insured proper infant nutrition, but the length of time it occurred varied among the different ethnic groups. Indians tended to breast feed for three to five years with supplemental solid food. Africans bound to slavery were encouraged to wean infants at about a year old, and the supplementary foods were often deficient in protein and had few vitamins, such as corn gruel and small bits of salt pork. Europeans tended to wean infants no later than two years of age, and breast milk was usually supplemented by soft foods such as cereal gruel or bread soaked in milk or water (Tannenbaum 2012: 73–75).

Children needed to be trained both cognitively and physically. "To the seventeenth-century mind, human beings were quite literally made, not born" (Calvert 1992: 19). Shaping the child into a proper human began with swaddling. In order to ensure that babies grew with straight legs and backs, they were bound with strips of linen, a process shared by Indians and Anglo-Americans. An Indian variant of the linen swaddling bundle created in Euro-American households was the cradleboard, infant carriers of leather and wood that were strapped on the back of adults. The idea was essentially the same—to create upright walking and erect adults by conditioning them as infants.

A straight and upright posture ensured, at least in European and American minds, demonstrating their distance from the other animals. Intellectual thought at the time emphasized three main things that separated humans from the other animals—speech, complex thought and reasoning, and upright and bipedal movement. In keeping with the thought that bipedality was a uniquely human trait, crawling on all fours was seen as "animalistic."

Swaddling usually lasted for three to six months, and the process had several possible impacts on well-being. For one, the infant was bound into an immobile state and could not stretch or move their limbs. Unlike diapers, which are changed several times a day, swaddling bands were complicated, multiple windings of linen and were likely changed far less regularly. The large number of recipes for salves and potions for diaper rash and other skin diseases found in the medical guides of the time support the notion that swaddling was not a hygienic practice.

Swaddling was common until the end of the eighteenth century when new ideas about child rearing emphasized that nature should run its course (Tannenbaum 2012: 73). Following swaddling, the child was often introduced to another common piece of furniture designed expressly for children, one that prevented crawling—the standing stool. It was essentially a round hole, often very snug, through which the child was placed and held upright. In addition to their function of keeping the child erect, they kept infants off cold and dirty floors and away from the dangers of fireplaces and other hazards. Standing stools were frequently followed by walking stools, also known as baby walkers. Unlike modern child walkers, they had no seat, but they did share the familiar set of upright supports on wheels that allow for motion. They ranged in design and construction from very simple to very ornate, the latter often having carved wood pieces.

There were few pieces of furniture designed specifically for children in the colonial Euro-American household, and most were associated with the idea of restrictive movement which shaped the growing infant. The cradle was one of those, and also served to foster erect posture and upright movement. Most cradles prior to the mid-1800s were built of wood and were long and narrow to accommodate the swaddled child. They were often covered with a cloth, and the high sides and ends of the cradle, combined with the cloth, kept cold drafts from reaching the infant.

Ensuring that children grew up to match the expectations of adult stature and erect posture was only one aspect of raising children in the colonial period. From birth until about age five, children were faced with a number of nutritional challenges and infectious diseases. Childhood mortality was high, about 25 percent prior to the age of five, with rates as high as 50 percent for enslaved Africans (Tannenbaum 2012: 69). Gastrointestinal disorders and intestinal parasites were common especially after weaning. Among the common infectious diseases children were afflicted with were diphtheria, scarlet fever, measles, and whooping cough. High rates of mortality for children under the age of five would remain until advances in hygiene and medical care occurred about 1850.

Women Caring for Themselves

A central part of women's ability to provide care for their families was for them to be healthy themselves. Nutrition and infectious disease were certainly important issues for colonial women, but a lot of emphasis was also placed on sexuality and reproduction. After all, two-thirds of a woman's reproductive years could be spent either pregnant or breast feeding children (Tannenbaum 2012: 58). Childbirth was an extremely frightening event as maternal mortality was quite high until the nineteenth century. Among Anglo-American women, about 20 percent died as a result of childbirth (Demos 1970: 131). The mortality rates due to childbirth were even higher for those of African descent who were bound to slavery.

Sex and pregnancy were seen in the seventeenth and eighteenth centuries as healthy and good for several reasons. Women's humours ran cold, and regular sexual activity was thought to add "heat" and keep them healthy. It was also thought that regular sexual activity prevented the accumulation of menstrual blood. Menstruation was seen in early colonial times as nature's way of purging poisonous humours from the body; suppressed or obstructed menses were a sign of poor health.

A missed menstrual period was called "taking a cold," a phrase that reflected the Galenic concept that menstrual blood was a "hot" humour, and its absence reflected a cold humour. Menstruation, childbearing, fertility, and reproductive health were attended to by communities of women. Men had no place in any of these areas of knowledge until about the mid-nineteenth century when a number of shifts in thinking and technology brought men into the practice of childbirth as obstetricians (see Chapter 4).

The process of conception in the seventeenth and eighteenth centuries was murky at best. It was not clear whether males provided the entire structure of a child that was simply "planted" in the female womb, or if both men and women contributed parts of the structure. It seemed clear, however, that men contributed the "heat" that was essential for the structure (fetus) to grow. Another part of the murky understanding of reproduction was the recognition of pregnancy, which was complicated in the seventeenth and eighteenth centuries.

While the connection between suppression of menstruation (amenorrhea) and pregnancy was recognized, most people thought that there were other reasons why menses might be suppressed and signal an unhealthy state. Full recognition of pregnancy was generally placed on the first movement of the fetus, a time known as "quickening," which occurred in the third to fifth month of gestation. Thus, it was often not clear prior to quickening if a missed menstrual cycle was due to pregnancy or was a sign of illness.

The absence of a clear sign that amenorrhea was due to pregnancy brought concerns of health, and there were a number of medicines and practices, "emmenagogues" (agents that increase menstruation) that were known to assist in stimulating and maintaining the menstrual cycle. Many of these involved plants that were associated with restoring menstruation, a healthy condition, but there were also vigorous exercises, rubbings of the abdomen, bloodletting, douches, and baths. Among the drugs often used to stimulate menstruation were aloe (*Aloe barbadensis*), pennyroyal (*Hedeoma puegiodes*), madder (*Rubia tinctorum*), seneca snakeroot (*Polygala senega*), and either savin (*Juniperus sabina L.*) or red cedar (*Juniperus virginiana L.*). Many were known by Indians, and the knowledge of their attributes and administration came clearly from native healers.

The actual intent of women using these means of restoring menses is unclear. There is considerable evidence that, by at least the eighteenth century, the role of emmenagogues for contraception and abortion was well known. As Susan Klepp said, "Definitions of disease—obstructed menses, colds, rheumatism, even worms or internal parasites—along with a reticence in speaking or writing about private female topics have hidden the contraceptive and abortive technologies available to Pennsylvania women in the eighteenth and early nineteenth centuries" (Klepp 1994: 81).

Similarly, discussions among Africans skirted the issue of pregnancy and compounds used to treat missing menses and other females' complaints. Couched in conversations of illness caused by conjurers, one type of invasion of the body by animals was called "frogs in the stomach." The compounds recommended to remove a frog from the stomach, such as turpentine, sassafras, and asafetida (also asafoetida; *Ferula* sp.), are all known abortifacients (Hyatt 1970; Mathews 1992a; Wilkie 2003).

Domestic Medicine Handbooks

Beyond family knowledge and recipe books, there were also written sources on domestic medicine. There was a time, of course, in the early colonial period when any written information was difficult to access, but after the mid-eighteenth century, a number of publications were produced, often by physicians, in the form of do-it-yourself pamphlets and books available for consultation by laypersons. Those publications presented explanations of the symptoms and signs of disease, as well as explanations of common medical terminology.

Perhaps one of the earliest and certainly well-known written sources was William Buchan's *Domestic Medicine*. Originally published in Edinburgh in 1769, the first American edition was published in Philadelphia 26 years later (Buchan 1795; see also Buchan 1809). An immensely successful book, it was revised and republished in America and Britain several times. Buchan felt that physicians had an obligation to provide the public with medical knowledge, especially with regard to prevention rather than care of acquired conditions.

Buchan, a physician himself, emphasized a balance between the separate roles of educating the public but preserving the role of specialists: "We do not mean that every man should become a physician. This would be an attempt as ridiculous as it is impossible. All we plead for is, that men of sense and learning should be so far acquainted with the general principles of Medicine, as to be in a condition to derive from it some of those advantages with which it is fraught; and at the same time to guard themselves against the destructive influences of Ignorance, Superstition, and Quackery" (Buchan 1772: xix).

Buchan's text was organized topically, with chapter headings such as "Of Customary Evacuations," and "Of the Passions," and "Of Diseases." Consider the following passage from "Of the Passions": "It is not indeed always in our power to prevent being angry; but we may surely avoid harbouring resentment in our breast. Resentment preys upon the mind, and occasions the most obstinate chronical disorders, which gradually waste the constitution. Nothing shows true greatness of mind more than to forgive injuries: It promotes the peace of society, and greatly conduces to our own ease, health, and felicity" (Buchan 1772: 139).

Another popular hero of domestic medicine texts was J. C. Gunn, whose *Domestic Medicine, or Poor Man's Friend* graced many a family's bookshelf. Published first in Knoxville in 1830, by 1870 after it had reached its 100th edition, it was renamed Gunn's *New Family Physician; or Home Book of Health*. Gunn's purpose was to bring medical knowledge to people by promoting common sense and using common language. It was organized in much the same way as Buchan's text, topically by disorder or complaint. His description of Dysentery or Flux is very visual: "This disease is always accompanied with *Tenesmus,* or a constant desire to go to stool, without being able to pass much of any thing from the bowels, excepting a *bloody kind of mucus*—which resembles that generally scraped from the entrails of a hog. These desires to go to stool, are usually accompanied with *severe griping,* and also with *some fever*" (Gunn 1830: 190).

Several other texts appeared with similar messages to those of Buchan and Gunn, such as Benezet's *The Family Physician* (1826), Cooper's *Treatise of Domestic Medicine* (1824), Ewell's *American Family Physician* (1824), Matthews's *Treatise on Domestic Medicine* (1848), and Ruble's *The American Medical Guide for the Use of Families* (1810). What all shared was that the author was a physician and that one of their central goals was to educate domestic readers in medicine so they would know to call in a doctor for serious problems.

Domestic health care texts, however, were not limited to those written by physicians. There was a countermovement that stressed that domestic health care could be accomplished just fine by nonphysicians. One of the most long-lived and influential of such texts was *Primitive Physick* by the well-known Methodist preacher, John Wesley. Published first in London in

1747, it was reprinted in Philadelphia in 1764 and continued to be reprinted in America throughout the nineteenth century (Wesley 1764). Wesley said his book made it possible to have a physician in the home without a fee by knowing what cure was needed for a particular symptom. His cures were mostly herbal and provided simple, safe medicines without some of the harsh ingredients in pharmaceutical compounds such as mercury or opium (Blake 1977).

Lay Practitioners

Lay practitioners provided the most affordable health care outside of family and friends to seventeenth- and eighteenth-century colonists. Their services were acknowledged through payments ranging from exchange of services, to presentation of goods, to monetary payment. Lay practitioners included midwives, women who were able to turn their household skills into paid medical practice ("doctoresses" or "doctor women"; Tannenbaum 2002), and clerics. For the most part, lay practitioners were recognized for their skills and experience, but they often did not receive informal training through internships.

Midwives

The most familiar lay practitioners were midwives. Midwives are generally associated with providing assistance in the process of giving birth, although their skills and assistance went far beyond that. They were engaged in all aspects of reproductive health from preconception through the early years of child care. Midwives linked communities of women to each other, often through multiple generations, and until the twentieth century were the main consultants in matters of female health, especially reproductive health. With the exception of middle- to upper-class women living in urban settings, most women were assisted in birth, and in matters of mothering, from their female relatives, close friends, and from a midwife. Midwives were also deeply spiritual and their spirituality, combined with their traditional approaches to childbirth and reproductive health, maintained a healthy continuance of home health care.

Women were typically "called" to midwifery after they had been mothers themselves, and most went through an apprenticeship to an older, established midwife. Although there were published guides to midwifery, such as Jane Sharp's *Midwife's Book* (1671, 1725), it seems that most midwives learned their trade through experience (and survival) as mothers of many children. Thus, most were middle-aged or older during their practicing years.

With such a wide range of skills and applications, the tool kit of a midwife could be rather extensive. Most midwives prior to the late 1800s made their own salves, lotions, and elixirs; herbs and other plants were used, and often infused with alcohol. Animal remedies were also employed, such as gelatin made from calves feet, and beef broths and teas.

> Now for a cough, a bad cough, we would use those hog-hoof teas. Now my mother made us use that tea. My father killed hogs for our pork meat all the time and we would save the hoof off the hog feet just like we would anything else for winter teas and salves. They used to use the inside of an eggshell, that little thin piece. I wish I could remember what they did with that. They used to use that in some kind of tea too. (Onnie Lee Logan, an African American midwife as told to Katherine Clark, Logan 1989: 61)

Birth in the early colonial days was a woman's affair, and men generally were not present for the event (Leavitt 1986). The midwife would attend the birth once she was called, usually after the mother reported that the contractions were felt. She was joined by other women as it was the common experience that "women attended other women in their confinements" (Leavitt 1986: 37). During the early stages of contractions, the midwife would often prepare the woman's body for the transformation of birth by anointing her with oils, braiding her hair, powdering her, and sprinkling sweet smelling waters on her body (Mongeau 1985).

Most midwives were skilled at mitigating the many possible complications that could occur during childbirth, such as turning the child in the womb, and providing medicines that would hasten labor. There were few tools used by midwives in the birth event, unlike the large number of devices used by trained obstetricians. One of the most recognized material manifestations of the midwife's kit was the birthing stool or chair (Figure 2.2), which provided a place for the mother to sit, for gravity to assist in the birth, and for the midwife to have access to the birth canal.

> There are so many women that want to have babies in that sitting position. It's not unusual. It feels good. The mother gets more relief. . . . I have delivered babies on purpose on their knees like that with a chair like this here. Because that makes her comfortable. I had mine on my knees. It's whatever makes you comfortable. I will do that for a

home delivery because that's the purpose of home delivery. That's the privilege of staying home. (Onnie Lee Logan, an African American midwife, as told to Katherine Clark [Logan 1989: 152])

Oils and massages might be used to ease the delivery and soften the perineum (the area between the anus and the vulva). Grease could be used to lubricate the birth canal. Herbal teas might be used to stimulate contractions.

The extension of the duties and skills of a midwife went far beyond the process of birth, and early child care included issues of spirituality. Conjuring, both to discern the cause of illness or health problems, as well as to

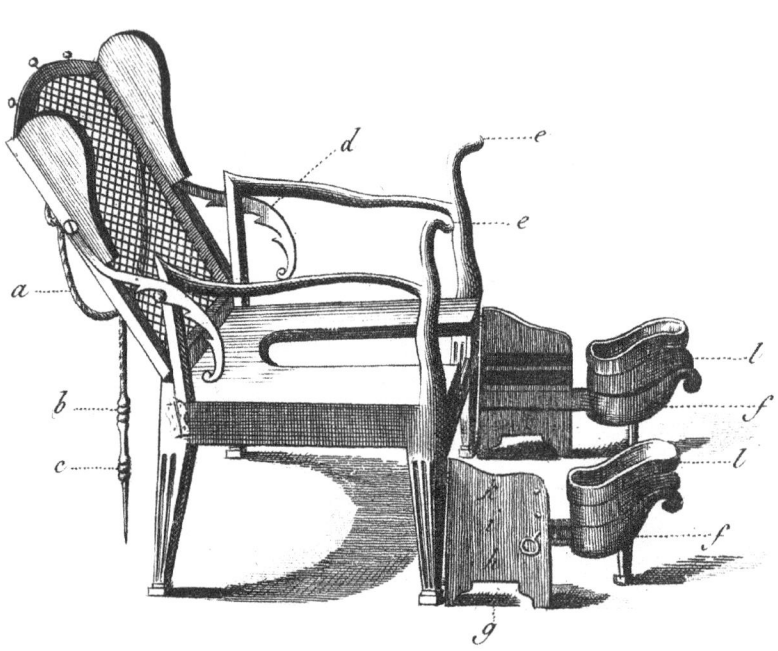

Figure 2.2. Parturition chair described by G. G. Stein in *L'Art d'Accoucher*, Paris 1804, figure 9 Wellcome Images. This file comes from Science Museum Group, in the United Kingdom. Refer to Wellcome blog post (archive, https://commons.wikimedia.org/wiki/File:Parturition_chair_Wellcome_M0012293.jpg).

bring about results, was routinely practiced by midwives (Mathews 1992a, 1992b; Schwartz 2006; Wilkie 2003). Another was in the practice of restoring menstruation. As noted previously, the absence of menstruation was not necessarily linked to pregnancy, and could be interpreted as a health issue. Midwives administered a number of different plants and other compounds to restore menstruation (emmenagogues). The problem was that those emmenagogues caused abortions.

The legal status of abortion was often unclear in the seventeenth century (Klepp 1994; Tannenbaum 2002). If "quickening" was not recognized, any intervention that caused the loss of the fetus, such as restoring menstruation, was not recognized as an abortion. In fact, the first English statute on abortion in 1623 defined criminal abortion as one that takes place after quickening. No American prosecutions explicitly for abortion occurred until the 1740s (Tannenbaum 2002: 39). However, the more it was recognized that the emmenagogues administered to restore menstruation also caused abortions, the more midwives fell subject to criticism.

Doctoresses

Women were not limited to practicing as midwives. Doctoresses were skilled professionals who differed from midwives in several ways. They did not center their attention solely on female medical issues, but extended their care to both women and men. They generally did not look after cases related to childbirth, but provided their services to patients with chronic and/or contagious illnesses, often for long-term periods. Some provided care within their homes around the clock, and in addition to medical care, provided food and drink, and bathing. They were paid fairly significant sums, well beyond the simple fees or goods that were provided to midwives. Some did surgery, although the extent and depth of their surgical practices are unclear. The training of doctoresses is unfortunately not very well documented.

The practice of a doctoress was thus much more like that of a male physician. Their clientele, their fees, their focus largely on issues that extended beyond "female complaints" differentiated them from other female health practitioners. Similar to midwives, doctoresses were sometimes seen as unwelcome competitors by many male physicians (Tannenbaum 2002). Because of the middle ground that doctoresses had between women whose medical practices were largely in the household or with nearby neighbors, and male physicians, they were often recipients of criticism.

By breaking beyond traditional female roles with a focus solely on family and neighbors' health, doctoresses were more likely than other female healers to face scrutiny and even prosecution. In fact, much of the available documentation regarding doctoresses is in the form of legal proceedings. Some of these were centered on malpractice, but they were more commonly in the form of accusations of witchcraft.

One example is Mary Hale who ran a smallpox hospital in Boston during the mid- to late seventeenth century (Tannenbaum 2002). She was a widow and her care of the sick provided her financial support. Mary Hale was accused of witchcraft in 1681 by a male boarder, Michael Smith. The accusation was that Hale had hoped that Smith would marry her granddaughter, and upon finding out that he was courting another woman, cast a spell on him and made him sick (Tannenbaum 2002: 126–127).

It was not the only case that involved Mary Hale. She had, the year earlier, in 1680, been an important witness in a case that involved a slave, Zanckey, who had become ill. The case largely involved past-due medical bills and money owed for labor. Zanckey had been sent to Hale's establishment with a diagnosis of smallpox, but the disease turned out to be syphilis (Tannenbaum 2002: 120–121). Hale was on good relations with two male practitioners and was able to work with them on curing Zanckey. She was awarded the past-due medical charges, and seems to have maintained good relationships with her male physician colleagues.

Clerics

Clerics and ministers also practiced medicine as a logical extension of their community service (Watson 1991). They were often highly educated, knew many of the individuals in a community, were well informed of medical events, and had access to medical books in their libraries. One of the most notable minister-physicians was Cotton Mather, who lived between 1663 and 1728. Mather was educated at Harvard University where he earned both a B.A. and an M.A. He was an avid reader of medical texts, a practitioner of medicine, and a writer of medical works. His best-known medical work was *The Angel of Bethesda,* written in the 1720s but unpublished until the twentieth century (Mather 1972).

Cotton Mather was elected as a Fellow to the Royal Society of London in 1713 for his scholarly work. His election provided him access to the society's written holdings, and there he found manuscripts describing smallpox variolation/inoculation as practiced in Turkey. He also knew of the practice through conversing with his African slave, Onesimus, who told him of practices in Africa to prevent smallpox. During a smallpox epidemic in 1721, he used his pulpit to deliver the method of preventing smallpox, hoping that doctors in attendance would employ it.

Only one doctor, Zabdiel Boylston, took up the practice. Many would agree that the implementation of inoculation was immensely successful in providing the patient with mild cases of smallpox; of the 247 inoculations he provided by early 1722, only 6 had died. It remained controversial, however, and for more than 20 years numerous voices opposed the process. With continuing evidence of the positive effect of inoculation, though, Boylston and Mather won their campaign to bring inoculation to America.

Semiformally Trained Practitioners

Medical practitioners in the seventeenth and eighteenth centuries in America who had training and/or experience beyond lay practitioners often did not have, or necessarily need, a medical degree. English medical practitioners belonged to three distinct groups: physicians, surgeons, and apothecaries. The most learned were university-trained physicians. Many attended either Oxford or Cambridge for a fourteen-year period, after which they received their Medical Doctorate. Those schools were only available to members of the Church of England, however. There was little practical experience during their training, and their education largely focused on theory. An even more celebrated medical school was the University of Edinburgh, which was nonreligious and thus had no restrictions on admission. It also offered an MD degree in just three years. Regardless of which school they attended, few of the Europeans who trained formally at university emigrated to America before 1750.

Apothecaries, Physicians, and Dentists

In early colonial America, the distinctions between physicians, surgeons, and apothecaries did not exist. Learned practitioners of medicine in the early colonies were usually educated men, many with no formal training. They were often wealthy, well-respected individuals. A good example is Landon Carter of Virginia. Carter was a large landowner whose tobacco plantation was home to his family and staffed by tenant farmers and slaves. He kept an extensive diary (Carter 1965) in which he describes his medical knowledge, mostly obtained from a large collection of medical books, and his use of herbal drugs, emetics, bloodletting, and purges to heal his family and others to whom he provided medical care.

Surgeons and apothecaries in America were generally trained by apprenticeship, and in many ways they were like other skilled trades. Young men often began apprenticeships in their teens and studied for about six or seven years. Students generally sought a practitioner with whom they could study, and they often lived with the family of their mentor. They were generally educated in basic literature and read extensively in their mentors' libraries. In many cases, they assisted in the compounding of medicines, dressed wounds, and performed bleeding and other day-to-day tasks of patient care.

Itinerant Medical Specialists

Another group of healers included itinerant physicians, healers, and surgeon-dentists. Benes (1990: 96) defines these as "medical itinerants [who] traveled and advertised speculatively in order to attract patients; they were distinguished from resident or established physicians, pharmacists, and midwives who were willing to travel to their patients' homes, some distance if necessary, but whose livelihood did not depend on a continuing infusion of new clients in new places." For most itinerants, their formal medical training was unclear, despite their universal use of the title "Dr." Certainly some of them based their qualifications on things like "formerly educated by my father" or being the "seventh son of a seventh son" or "a method acquired while living among the Indians" (Benes 1990: 101–106).

The earliest of these itinerants recorded in the American colonies was Dr. Sharp, a specialist from London, who advertised in the *Boston Gazette* in 1720 that he claimed to be able to heal cancered breasts, other cancerous tumors, leprosy, King's evil, scurvy, rheumatisms, and ulcers (Benes 1990: 97). Itinerant healers were numerous in the 1760s and 1770s, and the principal American seaports saw waves of oculists, aurists, surgeons, medical sellers, and surgeon-dentists. They came principally from England, France, and Germany.

Among the more interesting of the colonial itinerants was Dr. James Graham who came to America in 1770. He was a self-titled "oculist and aurist" (eye and ear doctor), but also advertised his skills as healing female complaints, cancers, old sores, and scorbutic ulcers. He was also well known for use of electrical cures and sex therapy. A prototype of his *Grand State Celestial Bed* was constructed in America before he returned to England near the beginning of the Revolutionary War.

Graham's final electrified, magnetic Celestial Bed in the Temple of Hymen, located in London, was domed by musical automata, flowers, and a pair of live turtle doves. Many, so it is said, experienced its tilted frame suspended above a multitude of magnets, which put couples in the best position to conceive, and whose movements set off organ music and celestial sounds accompanied by ethereal odors that wafted down from the dome above the bed. Sadly, there are no known illustrations of the bed except the cartoon reconstruction done by Tim Hunkin (2004). Graham was finally recognized as a charlatan, however, and he died in poverty in 1794.

Dental problems were commonplace in early colonial America. There were numerous itinerant dentists, but many other practitioners such as blacksmiths, general surgeons, and even laypeople extracted teeth. The first traveling dentist to arrive in America was John Baker, who came to Boston in January of 1767 (Benes 1990: 102; Weinberger 1948). He treated thousands of people and, over two decades, traveled to many places, among them Annapolis, Baltimore, Williamsburg, New York, Philadelphia, and Lancaster. Itinerant dental practitioners represented about 90 percent of those active in dentistry before 1800, a fact that slowly began to change after 1820 as more travel routes were repeated and fixed practices became common (Weinberger 1948).

A dentist's tool kit contained a number of items. One of the most common tools used was an extraction instrument called a key, which featured a shaft with a hooked end and a perpendicular wooden handle (Figure 2.3). It provided extra leverage as the person performing the extraction turned the key whose hook was attached to the tooth. George Washington's favorite dentist was John Greenwood who began as a lay practitioner. Greenwood's father practiced as a dentist in Boston, but was also a skilled maker of mathematical instruments. Following a career in the militia, John Greenwood worked as a dentist, made dentures, and designed and built one of the first dental drills. The drill was powered by a foot pedal, and the prototype was made from his mother's spinning wheel. Specialized furniture was also part of the dentist's tool kit, especially the dentist's chair which positioned the patient so that the mouth was at the correct angle.

Despite more sedentary dental practices, traveling dentists persisted well into the twentieth century, and one of the most flamboyant of those was Dr. Edgar Randolph Parker, better known as Dr. Painless Parker. He was born in Canada, and his first dentistry involved traveling throughout Canada transported by a buckboard. Parker moved to Brooklyn, New York, near the turn of the century and established an office practice, but throughout his 59-year career, he returned frequently to traveling dentistry.

At one point, after moving to the West Coast, Parker established the

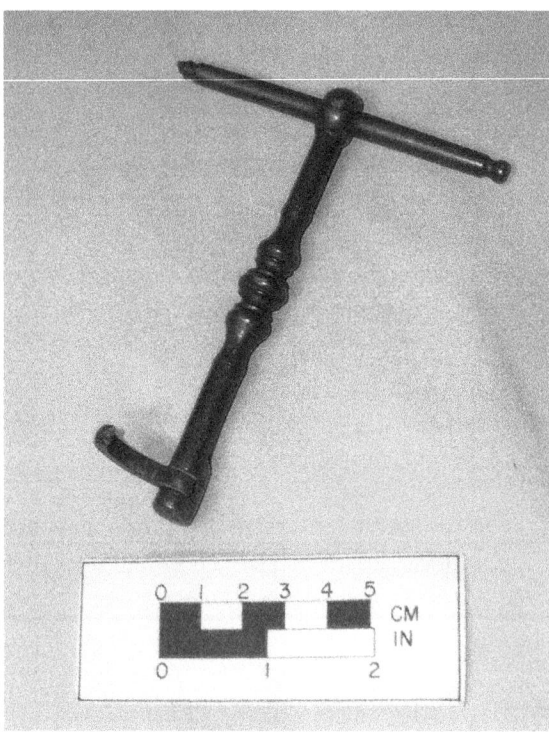

Figure 2.3. Dentist's key. Photographed by the author at the Country Doctor Museum, Bailey, NC.

Parker Dental Circus, complete with a bandstand imitating a gaping open mouth—where the band seemed at any moment about to be eaten—a tattooed lady, and a large tent staffed by four dentists, four doctors, four occultists, and Painless Parker throwing coins while riding an East Indian pachyderm (Armstrong and Armstrong 1997: 181). Parker operated 28 dental offices on the West Coast toward the end of his life, but he remained a showman—an article published in *Colliers* magazine the year he died at 80 has him adorned in a top hat with a necklace of 357 human teeth that he removed in one day near Poughkeepsie, New York.

* * *

Written documents form the bulk of the information about the role of women in the household with regard to healing and well-being. Clearly, those documents are both biased and partial sources. Europeans would have been the most literate women in the early colonies; consequently, the information presented regarding those of African or Indian descent would be both filtered and likely misinterpreted. Literate men of social standing would also have presented a filtered view of their role and that of others in the healing process. In the documentary discussions, men are rarely, if ever, mentioned. Certainly any archaeological information that could be brought to bear on the issue would be welcome.

II

Growing Pains

The Emergence of Specialized Medicine, 1750–1850

3

The Rise of Institutional Care

> In preindustrial society the family provided not only the basic necessities of life, but assumed responsibility as well for educating children, caring for the aged and infirm, and for supporting dependent members. The separation of home from the workplace—a characteristic of nineteenth-century industrial society where labor was often centralized in factories and other industrial or commercial workplaces—led to the privatization of family life.... The weakening of traditional means of socialization within the family and control by the family ultimately fostered the creation of public structures to take its place.
>
> (Grob 1994: 24)

America prior to 1750 was largely a rural country with an economy centered on the artisan system of labor, one which relied heavily on generational continuity in occupation, and with internship as a form of learning. The artisans produced an item from start to finish, usually in a shop adjacent to their homes. For instance, a shoemaker would fit the customer and then make the shoes at his shop on the same property. By 1750, a national and international marketplace was emerging with a system of wage labor. The journeyman artisan system was being undermined by the emergence of mercantile capitalism and specialized laborers. Separate parts of the shoemaking process were sent out to specialists.

The separation of home and workplace, as noted by Grob above, combined with a declining artisan economy, served to undermine family cohesion. The impact of an economy based around wage labor was felt earliest and most dramatically in the cities. Urbanization, while definitely in place, was still a minor part of the American settlement pattern; in 1790, there were only six major cities and only 3.35 percent of the population lived in them, roughly 8,000 residents. Between 1800 and 1850 there was a 1,000 percent increase in population (Curry 1981). By 1850, there were 85 urban centers and they contained 12.5 percent of the population; New York alone held half a million people (Grob 1994: 23). Much of the population growth came through immigration, and immigration was frequently linked both to high mobility and to poverty. Between 1820 and 1860 over five million immigrants came to America (Katz 1986).

With so many people living in urban environments, the number of laborers exceeded the available labor much of the time, and the vagaries of wage labor had some consequences for out of work laborers. Work was often temporary, seasonal, and offered low wages (Katz 1986). Much of the unskilled labor took place outdoors in agriculture, construction, and unloading ships. Frequent periods with no work ensured that laborers could not save money to cushion those out-of-work times. There were also limitations on how far away one could work as most people could not afford transportation and had to work within walking distance of their jobs. Competition for jobs left employers with the option, often embraced, of reducing wages.

Matthew Carey, an influential Philadelphia publisher and economist, gave an example of the wage problem using figures from the Board of Canal Commissioners (Carey 1828). Assuming that work was always available, a male laborer could earn $12 per month for 10 months and $5 per month for 2 months. His wife's annual income would be $13, and their total yearly income would be $143 ($3,883 in 2020 currency). Their budget, if modest, would include annual expenses of $26 for rent, $65.20 for food, $26 for adult clothes, and $16 to provide clothing for two children. Add to that some meager expenses for fuel and other necessities, and the necessary income required to survive for a year was $145.74 ($3,958 in 2020 currency). Thus, poverty became commonplace, and the family structure was often eroded further by the necessity of turning to labor distant from home and/or dangerous.

Massive growth in places like New York and Philadelphia challenged the material demands of housing and sanitation, as well as the immune systems of the inhabitants. Constant ship traffic meant both a steady supply of infected passengers and new supplies of those susceptible to infectious diseases already present. Vectored diseases such as malaria and yellow fever were facilitated by ship traffic in the ports of Charleston, New York, and Philadelphia. Quarantine was no small part of the package of ship fevers, and special locations and facilities (pest houses) were developed to provide ships of infected passengers with a place of transition.

Massive population growth, increased mercantilism, and faster migration and mobility, all facilitated the breakdown of family structure and

America's new social and economic stratification. Poverty became a mainstay in the lives of many, as did isolation. And so, institutions arose to provide help in caring for people. State hospitals and almshouses were places for those who could not afford medical care, and for the mad. Nonetheless, placement into an institution was largely reserved for impoverished urban orphans, the elderly, homeless, and chronically ill. Everyone agreed that medical care in the patient's home was best, with a central focus on family, relatives, and friends. However, not everyone had a choice.

Risky Trades

Coincident with the rise of wage labor, separation of home and workplace, urban growth, and poverty, was increased risk of health hazards in the workplace. Labor organizers as early as the 1700s in America realized that occupational hazards could negatively influence a person's health, perhaps as seriously as with an early death. Many occupations carried some risk of harm in the long term, but others had their own hazards unique to them. As examples, one could cite violence and sexually transmitted diseases as more of a risk for pirates and sex workers; or famine, disease, and trauma in military service or law enforcement; or respiratory diseases in mining; or infectious disease transmission as a physician. The list could certainly be much longer, but I limit my discussion here to the maritime trades and sex work, their consequences for health and well-being, and their contribution to the necessity of institutional care.

Maritime Trades

From the earliest days of the colonial experience, the movement of goods and people was carried out primarily by ships. It was well into the nineteenth century before any appreciable mercantile transport was conducted outside of the aquatic realm, and even then oceanic and riverine transportation remained important. The physical labor required of sailors was immense and the hazards of loading ships, scaling masts, and maintaining the ship were constant and dangerous.

The cargo being transported could seriously injure a sailor if it fell on him. Common transport containers were wooden barrels which could easily be tipped over and roll into a person. Stormy weather and rough seas could wash sailors over the edge, or even worse, doom a ship to sinking or going aground. Like any confined population, if an illness broke out while at sea (which happened on the American luxury passenger liner *Diamond Princess* and many other cruise ships during the Covid-19 pandemic), likely everyone was going to succumb to it.

Whaling carried additional hazards. Whales were hunted from small boats that ventured into a pod of whales and had to be close enough for a harpooner to lodge the harpoon into the whale. Wounded whales could come after the boats, or sailors could get tangled in the harpoon lines. Processing whales carried its own dangers with shipboard fires, hot oil being foremost among them. Some ships carried physicians, but more frequently the person who served as a medical consultant had rudimentary training.

Maritime voyages were lengthy affairs, often nine or ten months long, and much of the available food and water was stowed on the ship and meant to last that length of time. Dietary deficiencies that led to diseases such as scurvy were common, and the nutritional content of much of the food was often questionable. Scurvy results from a deficiency of vitamin C, and the most abundant sources, fresh fruit and vegetables, were both in short supply on long voyages.

Recognizing the importance and need for medical care for the maritime trades, many of the earliest hospitals were underwritten by an insurance fund to provide medical care for sailors on American vessels (Rosenberg 1987: 33). Merchant seamen were required to contribute to the fund (20 cents per month) in order to stabilize funds for possible hospitalization. In fact, substantial portions of the revenue for private hospitals came from employees of the maritime trades. For example, about half of the paying customers between 1833 and 1850 in New Haven Hospital were seamen. In Boston, the first hospital was one established by the government exclusively for seamen; Massachusetts General Hospital came later.

The ultimate risky maritime danger was piracy, which combined the hazards of the maritime trades listed above with those of armed conflict and illegality. A marvelous example of early eighteenth-century maritime medicine is presented in the excavation and analysis of the *Queen Anne's Revenge* (*QAR*), the flagship of Edward Thatch, better known as Blackbeard. Blackbeard captured the *QAR* from the French in 1717 as it was transporting 516 slaves across the Middle Passage, accompanied by three surgeons and a surgeon's assistant.

Most of the slaves and crew were set ashore, but ten Frenchmen and the surgeons were retained by Blackbeard and returned to France only after the *QAR* was grounded on a sandbar in Beaufort Inlet about June 10, 1718, in North Carolina. The shipwreck was discovered on November 22, 1996,

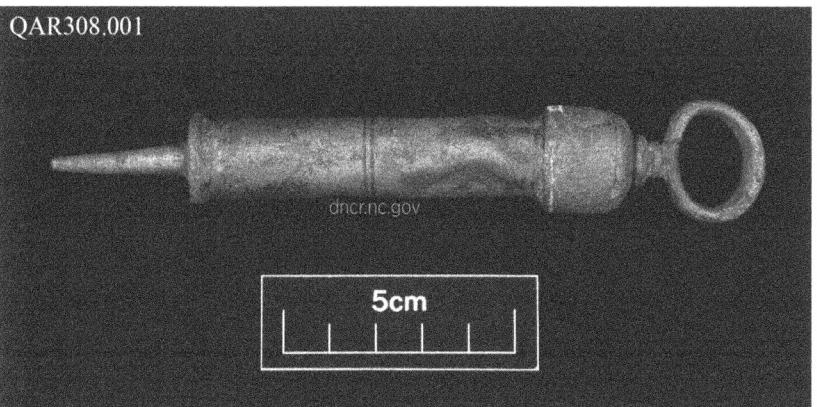

Figure 3.1. Urethral syringe recovered from the ship *Queen Anne's Revenge*. Image courtesy of North Carolina Department of Natural and Cultural Resources.

and excavation and conservation of the artifacts are currently under way. The medical artifacts recovered to date provide a glimpse into the medical needs and care of sailors in the early eighteenth century.

Among the medical artifacts recovered from the wreck were a mortar and pestle for grinding medicinal compounds; ceramic galley pots (and apothecary jars) filled with unguents, salves, balms, and potions; a pewter urethral syringe with a Paris trademark; two sets of nesting weights, probably used to measure compounds; two pairs of brass set screws, presumably used in a screw tourniquet; a pump clyster; and a crushed pewter porringer, probably used for bleeding. These are all discussed in detail and given context by Linda Carnes-McNaughton (2016; see also Wilde-Ramsing and Carnes-McNaughton 2018).

The urethral syringe is especially interesting (Figure 3.1). Urethral syringes were used for a number of purposes, including to relieve stoppages due to bladder stones and for the insertion of mercury, which was used to treat syphilis. Indeed, once artifact conservation of the syringe was completed, chemical analysis of the inside of the syringe showed that it contained mercury. Pump clysters were used to deliver medical enemas for relief of blockages, to cleanse the colon, and to inject medicines which could be absorbed more quickly (see Carnes-McNaughton 2016: Figure 13, for a wonderful view of a clyster being used).

In short, a number of hazards awaited those in the maritime trades. The fact that early on an insurance plan was developed for seamen, and the fact the earliest hospital in Boston was dedicated to providing medical assistance for them, serves testament to the dangers they faced medically.

Sex Work

Women who worked in the sex trade faced a number of health concerns. Foremost among them were sexually transmitted diseases, but their work also often placed them in danger of physical violence. Syphilis was among the common sexually transmitted diseases, and until the discovery of penicillin by Alexander Fleming in 1928, one of the standard treatments for syphilis was large doses of mercury. Mercury had several undesirable side effects, though, such as nausea, vomiting, and tooth loss. Consequently, doctors often recommended other treatments, none of them very effective. In severe cases of sexually transmitted disease, those where the infection left visual signs, it placed disfigured women without a source of income and into poverty. Many sex workers subsequently ended up in almshouses.

Another set of health hazards for those in the sex trade were pregnancy and childbirth. Women involved in sex work generally did not have the family structure to adequately raise a child, and their pregnancy often resulted in the entry to an almshouse to give birth. Childbirth was dangerous for any woman in colonial America, but combined with sexually transmitted infections, the risks were even higher. Children born in almshouses also suffered; one in six children in Philadelphia almshouses died within a few days of birth (Lyons 2006: 263). While a somewhat alarming percentage, examination of the juvenile skeletons from the Highland Park skeletal collection (Monroe County Poorhouse) showed that 40 percent died before the age of one; written documents for the poorhouse indicate that a slightly larger percentage (45 percent) died before age one (Higgins and Sirianni 1995: 128).

The illicit nature of the sex trade, and the stigmatization associated with it, combined with the consequences of sex work discussed above, could suggest a rather unsavory life. Yet there are several incorrect assumptions about sex work. A primary one is that women only entered the sex trade when they had no other choice (Wood 1993). There is plenty of evidence that the choice of women to enter into sex work was often about agency— women made decisions within the constraints placed on the actors that allowed them to control their lives. There are many documents written by women who make it clear that they consciously chose to sell sexual favors. For one thing, the money for a nineteenth-century woman working in a brothel was about ten times more than other available work (recall the $13 annual income for a woman in Mathew Carey's estimates).

A number of archaeological investigations at the sites of known brothels have contributed valuable insights into the lives of those engaged in the sex industry, both providers and clients.

Life in a brothel certainly had mixed issues. On the one hand, appearance was important. The furnishings and ambience of the establishment lubricated the attendance of its clientele. Clothing, jewelry, and other objects of personal adornment were often well represented in the archaeological deposits of brothels, a situation generally not true of other neighboring households. The culinary entertainment of the guests required fine presentation and ingredients, with variance given the class the brothel primarily served.

On the other hand, douching syringes and compounds, glass breast shields, and portable urinals provide supporting evidence that venereal diseases and pregnancy were risky consequences of the sex trade. For instance, the Padelford privy in Boston (also called the Endicott Street privy) was associated with a brothel in operation between 1853 and 1870. It contained 30 glass syringes that were likely used for vaginal douching (an established hygienic practice at the time), and glass breast shields used by women who were nursing.

Two neighborhoods in Washington, DC, were known for sex work, and archaeological excavations have occurred in each. The Island was an area separated from the rest of Washington by the Washington Canal and the Potomac River. The Island now includes the National Mall, and to the south of the Mall, several blocks of government office buildings. The other neighborhood known for sex work was called Hooker's Division, north of the Island. It is now at the west end of the Federal Triangle and Constitution Avenue.

Mary Ann Hall owned one of the most lavish and well-known brothels in Washington, DC. It was a high-class bawdy house, and was listed as a class 1 bawdy house in the 1864 provost marshall's report, which indicated there were 18 sex workers living there (USACE 1864–1865). Located at 349 Maryland Avenue on the Island, the remains of her property came back into light in 1997 when the location of her former house became part of the property for the planned National Museum of the American Indian. Artifacts such as flowerpot sherds and lamp-chimney glass, suggesting attention to decor and working at night, were more abundant at the brothel than in neighboring family households. Also more abundant than family households were clothing artifacts like buttons and shoes, although there were few personal items like mirrors or jewelry.

White ironstone dishes and porcelain tablewares at Mary Ann Hall's served specialty foods. Faunal remains included wild birds, turtle, and fish, which were accompanied by high to medium cuts of mutton, goat, beef, and pork; chickens (laying hens) were also kept on the property (Yamin and Seifert 2019: 64). Neighboring family households enjoyed far less lavish foods, mostly chicken and pork. A preferred beverage was champagne, and several foil bottle seals indicate the preferred brand was Piper Heidsieck of Reims, France (Yamin and Seifert 2019: 65). Even the plant foods consumed at Mary Ann Hall's brothel were exotic, and included raspberry, strawberry, fig, grape, peach, walnut, and coconut. Again, neighboring households had less-varied plant food remains (Seifert and Balicki 2005).

Archaeological data for sex work in Washington, DC, indicate that there was a class difference among brothels, and presumably among clients of those houses as well. Mary Ann Hall's class 1 brothel had numerous employees. Other bawdy houses were less lavish and generally had fewer employees. Archaeological investigations of brothels located in Hooker's Division Squares 257 and 258 in 1990 yielded artifacts from two brothels. They provide a comparative base for Hall's lavish house. Kitchen artifacts were frequent in the Hall's archaeological materials (83 percent), as compared to the more meager frequency (50 percent) from the Hooker's Division brothels (Seifert and Balicki 2005: 63). Ironstone and porcelain tableware were far more fancy and expensive at Hall's compared to the Hooker's Division brothels.

Sex work was common in nineteenth-century New York City as well. At least 200 brothels operated in New York in the 1820s, a number that grew to 600 by 1870 (Gilfoyle 1992: 31). A center of the sex trade in the 1830s and 1840s was the Five Points region (later Lower Manhattan), a notorious tenement slum. Between about 1830 and 1910, Five Points was a center of immigrant housing, violent crime, squalid living conditions, poverty, and disease. The living conditions were so awful that a young journalist, Jacob Riis, recorded them in photographs. As most of the buildings had little natural or artificial light, his work was enabled by the newly developed flash photography, and presented in his landmark book, *How the Other Half Lives* (Riis 1890).

The residents of Five Points in the mid-nineteenth century had limited options for health care. While for some, disease and other issues of wellness could be treated by doctors, for most the cost of a physician was beyond their reach. Instead, they relied on dispensaries, charitable hospitals, apothecary shops, or home remedies. Archaeological excavations in the early 1990s were conducted on Block 160 at Foley Square in Lower Manhattan and they provide abundant evidence of how Five Points residents treated illness.

Numerous glass artifacts and bottles were recovered from the excavations, including soda and mineral bottles (n=59); "ethical" medicine vials or bottles, those physician-prescribed or those administered by an apothecary or dispensary (n=266); patent medicine bottles (n=51); and two female urinals and a nursing shield associated with the Orange (Baxter) Street brothel (Bonasera and Raymer 2001). The suite of glass artifacts indicates that a variety of medicinal compounds were used by the Five Points residents, and that implements focused on hygiene were part of the tool kit of wellness.

Sixty-four plant taxa were identified in Five Points; 34 of those taxa were used by professional medical practitioners and laymen during the nineteenth century (Bonasera and Raymer 2001). The two most common medicinal plants, jimsonweed (*Datura stramonium*) and wormseed (Jerusalem Oak [*Chenopodium ambrosoides*]), were found in abundance at the Five Points Block 160 site. Jimsonweed is a narcotic plant which causes hallucinations and can be toxic. The leaf was usually smoked as a treatment for asthma, although the leaves, flowers, and roots could be made into poultices and salves used topically for boils, swellings, and skin ulcers (Crellin and Philpott 1989; Krochmal and Krochmal 1973). Jimsonweed seeds were found in almost every feature at the site. Wormseed, true to its name, was used to treat intestinal worms by consuming a tonic made from its seeds. It was especially known for treating roundworms, an interesting fact since Reinhard (1998, see Chapter 6) found numerous roundworm eggs in privy feature deposits from Five Points.

Among the plants were twelve species that were considered medical panaceas, and were often consumed in tonics. Other plants used for medicinal purposes, including blackberry/raspberry, were consumed as teas made from the bark which treated diarrhea and were used as a blood purifier. Known cures of scurvy included four fruits, lettuce, and four herbaceous plants. Several plant species were known to treat skin conditions and ulcers, while others had broad spectra of treatment, including respiratory conditions, fever, nerves, headache, and sore throat. Some of the plants, including the herbaceous weeds, may have been prepared as home remedies.

Several trends were revealed from the analysis of Five Points Block 160. An increase in embossed medicine bottles in the 1840s and 1850s likely indicates an increase in patent medicine availability. There appear to be different patterns of the material medical culture of Irish Americans and

German-Polish Americans. Irish Americans appear to have used far more patent medicines, and mineral and soda water, the latter known to have widespread physical and psychological benefits. In general, the deposits of German-Polish Americans show far less use of medical vessels (Bonasera and Raymer 2001).

Archaeological investigations at Five Points Block 160 produced materials at one site, a privy at 10/12 Orange Street, that were much more lavish than surrounding properties. They were recovered from a stone-lined privy shaft located behind a tenement and dating after 1840. An 1843 legal document brought against John Donahue makes it clear that the site was one that hosted a brothel.

Among the materials recovered from there were a complete Chinese Export porcelain set of plates, tea and coffee cups, and a tea caddy (Yamin 1998, 2000, 2005; Yamin and Seifert 2019: 46). Alcohol was enjoyed by the residents as indicated by 100 wine bottles and 65 tumblers. The food remains indicate both expensive and less expensive meals, and the remains of veal, beef short loin, lamb, soft-shell clams, and salmon were not found in adjacent households. Nonetheless, most of the food remains indicate more pedestrian meals with cheaper cuts of meat—picnic hams, pork hocks, and inexpensive fish—that were likely served to the brothel residents on cheaper porcelain also found at the site.

The evidence recovered at 10/12 Orange Street gives a mixed picture of the lives of the residents there. A sewing box containing hooks, eyes, straight pins, a thimble, folding ruler, bobbins, and beads indicates sewing was one of the leisure activities of the women. Buttons and some bits of cloth are the only items of personal adornment, but also recovered were shoes, combs, hairbrush and toothbrush, and mirror fragments. Toys and children's tea sets indicate that children also resided in the house. A number of artifacts indicate some of the health issues faced at 10/12 Orange Street. Thirty-nine medicine bottles, almost all prescription and not patent medicines, likely indicate a physician served the residents. Two glass urinals were found, most likely used by women confined to bed with venereal disease, a well-known practice.

The Orange Street privy also contained evidence of one darker aspect of sex work, pregnancy and abortion. Unwanted pregnancies were common, and two laws were enacted in New York to protect the unborn child. The first, New York's 1829 abortion statute, held abortionists legally liable; it was a law designed to protect women (Hill 1993: 237). There were numerous abortionists at the time, many not physicians, and botched abortions frequently led to a woman's death. The 1845 New York Abortion Act went further to hold women who sought to terminate a pregnancy criminally liable as well.

The skeletons of two neonates and one fetus were discovered in the privy at 10/12 Orange Street. Two of the individuals were full-term infants who died about the time of birth, the third a fetus of 4.5–5 gestational months at the time of death (Crist 2005). Neither full-term infant has skeletal lesions that would suggest any infectious disease affected the individuals, nor was there any evidence of trauma. The fetal bones were too eroded and fragmentary to assess for lesions.

The skeletons were in distinct levels in the privy and were mixed with the skeletal remains of nonhuman animals (faunal remains). Historical documents mention the practice of disposing of the remains of deceased babies in privies. Whether or not the babies at 12 Orange Street were infanticides is unclear, but the practice was well known in the nineteenth century, as Lane described for Philadelphia: "Typically they had given birth alone, and then perhaps stuffed the infant's throat with a rag to keep it from crying out, or having gone to the privy, the only place in the home or boardinghouse where they might safely be alone had dropped it down, into the vault below, immediately on cutting the cord" (Lane 1997: 121). The act of concealment of the children in a privy at 12 Orange Street and in other hiding places serves testament to the desperate obstacles that women faced in the sex trade.

Institutional Care

Following the Revolutionary War, social reform movements in the larger northeastern urban areas were directed at the poor. While partially driven by genuine concerns about the impoverished segments of the population, they were also fueled by middle-class worries about social disorder, crime, and alcohol abuse. The initial social support systems were known as "outdoor relief," which provided either financial support or nonmonetary basic necessities such as food and fuel to indigents in their homes. Unfortunately, that system of outdoor relief didn't work very well, and the poor remained largely in the confines of urban centers.

Almshouses, established in the early 1800s, created a way to provide "indoor relief" by sending the needy to specific institutions that provided not only shelter, but also ancillary support such as health care. They were often built outside of town and in complexes that had other institutions on the same property, such as hospitals and penitentiaries. The number of "inmates" of almshouses fluctuated seasonally as work was available when the climate was favorable. Hospitals were a logical outgrowth of almshouse infirmaries which served a somewhat different purpose and were funded initially through different means.

Institutional care was not the preference of most people, but only those with sufficient economic means were likely to continue the early colonial practice of centering health care and economic livelihood within the home. Many people needed some social support system that would provide the basic needs of life. That realization led to the establishment of institutional health care, largely through almshouses and hospitals.

Almshouses

Almshouses, also known as poorhouses, workhouses, poor farms, and somewhat later as county homes, provided assistance for a number of conditions: addiction, mental and physical illness, injury, pregnancy, orphanhood, elder age, and disability (Wagner 2005; Warner 1894). They were not particularly pleasant places to be and they often represented the last resort for those who entered through their doors. As well, they served a somewhat murky purpose—at times their mission was one of assistance, but at other times it seemed more one of confinement. Nonetheless, in a harsh world with few options for meeting basic needs, almshouses served both as a necessary function of caring for the poor, and as a symbolic divide between those who were morally corrupt and those who were not.

Sentiments about institutional care in the form of almshouses arose partly through the English Poor Law of 1601 which expressed the principle that society had a corporate responsibility to care for the poor. Every American colony followed suit and passed laws that provided relief for the poor as long as the indigent could prove that they were legal residents in the community where they lived (Grob 1973: 7). The financial support was initially provided by special taxes by residents in the towns and/or neighborhoods to support their poor neighbors (Tannenbaum 2012: 194).

The first almshouse located in America was the Boston workhouse in 1664 (Rothman 2002: 39), and like many almshouses, it was modeled after those institutions of sixteenth-century Europe designed to confine the poor. Most of the early almshouses were located in port cities where the urban population swelled with immigrants. Although they were specifically designed to assist the poor, they primarily served only poor people of

European descent; seldom were Indians or Africans admitted through their doors.

Those who inhabited the almshouses were expected to work for their keep unless their health prevented labor. A general perception of almshouse residents was that they were lazy or corrupt individuals who brought their fate upon themselves through sexual depravity or drug abuse, and thus the general tenor of almshouses was much more one of punishment and containment than of relief and comfort (Quincy 1827: 26). There were often, in fact, many in the almshouse who were ill, either acutely or chronically.

Medical care was provided for those who sought shelter in the almshouse, but the large medical wards were often overcrowded, understaffed, and only provisionally equipped. Bathing was sporadic at best, as was the changing of bed linens. The food in almshouses was often insufficient in both quantity and nutrients—scurvy and other nutritional deficiency diseases were common (Rosenberg 1987: 16, 32). Visits by physicians were infrequent and much of the patient care was provided by those convalescing. In fact, it was not uncommon for women to gain experience nursing fellow patients and then remain as staff nurses for decades.

How sufficient or insufficient was the care provided to almshouse inhabitants? It is likely that almshouse records only report very general information, such as food quality, but not the health outcomes. There are two main sources that can be used to investigate the quality of life and wellness at almshouses: historical documents and human skeletal and dental remains. Both types of sources have positive and less-positive aspects. They are best used in conjunction with each other, as most reports of osteological analyses of almshouse cemeteries have done (for example, Grauer and McNamara 1995; Grauer et al. 1995, 2016; Higgins and Sirianni 1995; Higgins et al. 2002).

Historical records provide demographic data in the form of censuses and cemetery records, which can be used to assess trends in mortality. They can also indicate causes of death, at least proximate causes of death (pneumonia is a common secondary cause of death and often is not indicated as a proximate cause). Historical records of mortality for the nineteenth century are often uneven and sporadic. Death records were generally left up to the individual states; the first permanent national Death Registration Area (DRA) was established in 1900, and included only ten states and the District of Columbia (Haines 1998). Haines and colleagues (summarized in Haines 1998) assembled historical records to create a series of abridged life tables for mortality and life expectancy. Their research tells us that in 1850, across the United States, the life expectancy at age 20 (e_{20}) was short: 38.4 years for males and 39.8 for females (Haines 1998). Infant mortality, male and female combined, was 229 per 1,000 births.

Analysis of human burials offers the opportunity not only to directly observe some skeletal and dental markers of health insults, but also to compare skeletal lesions indicating disease and malnutrition with local contemporary death records. Skeletal and dental lesions unfortunately are often general indicators of health and cannot be used as indications of specific diseases. For example, periosteal reactions are one of these lesions that have numerous etiologies (causes). They are caused by inflammation adjacent to the outer membrane of bones, and while they may be associated with specific diseases, it is often not possible to delineate which one(s). They are also caused by injury and surgery, and thus while many people describe them under the category of infectious disease, infection is not the only cause.

Another general indicator is enamel hypoplasia, an indicator of metabolic stress and/or metabolic disruption. Hypoplasias are the result of improper enamel deposition with resulting furrows or linear rows of pits on the tooth (Hillson 1996). They occur during the growing years of the tooth and are not subject to skeletal remodeling as is the case for skeletal lesions. Thus, they permanently record a variety of insults during growth.

Several dietary deficiency diseases cause skeletal lesions, among them vitamin C deficiency (scurvy), vitamin D deficiency (rickets, osteomalacia), and anemia. Dietary deficiency diseases do not usually occur singly, but rather in combination with several nutrient deficiencies. Porotic hyperostosis results from an expansion of the red-blood-cell–producing marrow of the cranium. It is often attributed to iron-deficiency anemia (Ortner 2003), although that interpretation has been challenged by Walker and coworkers (2009) who argue a better etiology would be vitamin B12 deficiency. It is a condition experienced only by children; the diploic marrow turns over into fatty marrow after the juvenile years. The lesions are consequently remodeled throughout the lifetime, and although they often can be observed for years, absence of a lesion in an older adult does not necessarily indicate absence of anemia as a child.

Scurvy, which affects the quality of structural tissue (for example, blood vessels), results in hemorrhaging. The resulting lesions can be confused with porotic hyperostosis, but patterning of lesions and appearance enable distinguishing it sometimes. Rickets results in deformation of the weight-bearing bones due to insufficient maturation of the skeletal tissue.

The oral cavity also provides insight into diet and health. Carious lesions (cavities) are caused by frequent consumption of carbohydrates, which turn over into sugars. The resulting fermentation caused by bacteria leads to focal degradation of the enamel. If the lesions progress, the tooth and adjacent alveolar tissue (that which houses the teeth), generally become infected. Severe infections can result in death after prolonged pain and agony. In many cases, though, the affected teeth are lost premortem, and the alveolar bone eventually heals.

Archaeological and historical data from the Monroe County Poorhouse in New York State provide some insight into the health of almshouse residents. Monroe Poorhouse was in use from 1826 until the end of the Civil War. Analysis of historical records regarding the cause of death in almshouses in New York State often indicates that the leading cause of death was consumption (pulmonary tuberculosis), followed often by gastrointestinal illnesses. Historical data which can be used to contextualize the skeletal data come from the Brighton Town Clerk's Records on paupers and from census data and Mount Hope records for the general population of Rochester (Higgins et al. 2002).

Life expectancy in Rochester between 1853 and 1857 was slightly higher than that mentioned previously for 1850, 40.6 for males and 42.1 for females (Haines 1998). Infant mortality was also lower than the general United States; during the first year of life, infant mortality in Rochester was 132 per thousand (Haines 1998). The Rochester historical records (Brighton and Mt. Hope) indicate that consumption was the leading cause of death among adults aged 20–29 for females and 30–39 and 50–59 for males (Higgins et al. 2002: 168). The second and third main causes of death for adults were typhus and cholera. The picture was even more bleak for infants and children. They frequently suffered from consumption, gastrointestinal disorders, respiratory disorders, and childhood diseases. One half of children died within their first year of life.

At the Monroe County Poorhouse, historical records indicate that most juvenile deaths were due to consumption, 15–40 percent (ranges are used throughout this discussion because the data were presented in four age categories; see original data in Higgins and Sirianni 1995). Gastrointestinal infection was the second most frequent (15–24 percent; Higgins and Sirianni 1995). While often not specifically referenced in the death records, other historical records suggest that the gastrointestinal disease was cholera. Among adult women, the most frequent causes of death were also due to gastrointestinal infections and consumption.

The Highland Park Skeletal Collection contains 296 individuals (83 females, 118 males, 67 juveniles, and 28 individuals of unknown age and sex) who were patients at the Monroe County Poorhouse (Higgins and Sirianni 1995). Analysis of the skeletons buried in the Highland Park Cemetery shows a combination of prolonged illness and chronic diseases, such as tuberculosis and syphilis, but also several chronic episodes of childhood physiological stress, such as enamel hypoplasia and porotic hyperostosis.

In the Highland Park sample, moderate to severe periosteal reactions of the tibia were twice as frequent for adult males as females (20 males, 10 females; Higgins et al. 2002: 170). The higher frequency for males could be due to occupational risks, conflicts, chronic infections, and a number of other causes. Five of 27 juveniles (18.5 percent) experienced slight periosteal reactions but none that were moderate or severe, suggesting that the higher rate among adults was due to accumulated life experiences, including infectious disease. Children likely did not live long enough at the Monroe County Poorhouse to develop skeletal lesions such as periosteal reactions.

In the Highland Park skeletal sample, porotic hyperostosis was rare for adults; of 193 observable crania, only three had porotic hyperostosis (1.5 percent), one male and two females. Three out of 38 juveniles (7.9 percent) exhibited lesions of porotic hyperostosis. With regard to both juveniles and women, comparison of the death records for the Monroe Poorhouse and those for the 1850 general population suggest similar causes and frequencies of death. In addition, the skeletal and dental lesions showed no significant differences from the death records, suggesting that the death records are fairly accurate.

Dietary deficiency diseases were not the only health impact experienced by the almshouse residents. Chronic poor dental health, as demonstrated by dental and skeletal lesions in the female Highland Park sample, was abysmal. Individuals frequently had cavities (carious lesions; n=37%; percentages are all for adult teeth), plaque on their teeth (calculus; n=29%), or experienced tooth loss (n=23%) or periodontal disease (n=11%)(Higgins and Sirianni 1995). Sutter (1995) found very similar dental pathology frequencies for males (Sutter 1995). The dental data suggest that the poorhouse residents had a rather poor, likely high-carbohydrate, diet.

A source of comparative data for Highland Park is the Peoria City Cemetery. Peoria is the second-largest city in Illinois, and the cemetery was in use between 1842 and at least 1861 (Grauer et al. 2016). It did not specifically serve as the cemetery for an almshouse. The city cemetery was relocated about five miles away and outside the main city limits in 1877, and was named the Springdale Cemetery and Mausoleum. As the old cemetery fell into disrepair, some families disinterred and relocated the bodies of relatives to the newer, more posh facility; however, it is unclear how many were moved.

In 1910, a public library was built on the property of the original Peoria City Cemetery. Plans were made in 2009 to enlarge the library, and excavations were conducted to determine how significant an issue human burials were in those construction plans. The resulting 300 features resembling grave shafts resulted in a redesign of the planned construction footprint, which reduced the number of impacted graves; 86 individuals were removed and studied. Grauer and colleagues (2016) situated their analysis of the skeletons alongside historical Peoria censuses from 1860 and 1870, and an 1876 Death Report published in the *Peoria Daily Transcript*.

Infant mortality as indicated by both actual burials and historical records was high at the Peoria City Cemetery. Thirty of the 86 individuals recovered (36.1 percent) died before the age of one (Grauer et al. 2016). Historical records support that high mortality rate: for 1850 23.6 percent of individuals died before the age of one, as compared to 25 percent in 1860 and 22.7 percent in the 1872 Death Report. Both the census reports of 1860 and 1870, and the Death Report of 1872 indicate that one of the two most common causes of infant mortality was tuberculosis, with the other cause being cholera in 1860, scarlet fever in 1870, and severe diarrhea in 1872 (Grauer et al. 2016).

Skeletal and dental pathological lesions were fairly common at the Peoria City Cemetery. Periosteal reactions were observed for 19 percent of individuals; however, 25 percent of those who died before the age of three and were buried there exhibited periosteal reactions (Grauer et al. 2016). Porotic hyperostosis was observed for 19 percent of individuals, and enamel hypoplasia for 42 percent of individuals. Joint alterations (degenerative joint disease) were observed for 60 percent of the individuals. Healed fractures were observed for seven individuals (9 percent).

The suite of lesions observed suggests that individuals living in Peoria experienced rather hard and short lives in the mid-nineteenth century. They may also suggest that the frequencies of pathological lesions seen in the Highland Park Skeletal Collection are not particularly indicative of dramatic differences in health between the New York almshouse residents and the general population in Peoria.

Hospitals

Hospitals created a place where the "deserving and respectable poor" could find better care and institutional support than was offered by an almshouse. The hospital as we know it today, with paid physicians, paying clients, large clinical staff, and abundant specialized equipment did not emerge until the early twentieth century. Rather, early hospitals were a logical outgrowth of the almshouses, which were insufficient to provide the needs of staggering numbers of impoverished citizens.

Hospitals in the eighteenth and nineteenth centuries were initially modeled on the British system of private or "voluntary hospitals." Rather than being funded by the tax dollars that supported almshouses, they were funded by private donors, philanthropists who believed that "voluntary hospitals" would serve a number of important functions. The donors, also known as "subscribers," were stakeholders in the enterprise and thus held influence in several facets of hospital maintenance. Physicians in these hospitals were generally elite individuals, and following in the British model of charitable institutions, volunteered their services without pay.

The first true American hospital opened in Philadelphia in 1752 and was followed within 40 years by hospitals in New York and Boston (Tannenbaum 2012: 201). From the outset, hospitals distinguished themselves from almshouses through their requirement that they provided medical care for cases that could be cured. They did not admit patients with contagious, sexually transmitted, or terminal diseases. Most of those admitted had conditions that doctors felt could be cured, or were pregnant women, or those injured in accidents. Another exception was the "insane," whose care was entrusted to hospitals until the mid-nineteenth century when specialized care facilities were introduced.

One of those areas of influence held by subscribers was to provide recommendations for admission, most frequently done through a reference. The number of references that a subscriber could provide was dependent on the amount of money they contributed—annual subscribers of five dollars to the New York Dispensary could provide two references, and those who contributed fifty dollars could provide an unlimited number of references for life (Rosenberg 1987: 25). The person making the reference generally provided some statement supporting the moral character of the proposed patient, such as, "I have known Mrs. Milne since four or five years: and she is well known to Mrs. Jackson, my sister Mrs. Henry, to Mrs. [Buckley], and to many other ladies. I believe we can all testify that she is deserving, industrious, well-behaved and respectable" (Jackson 1853, cited in Rosenberg 1987: 25).

The admissions process to a hospital was thus comprised of multiple stages: first, an assessment of the curability of a condition, performed by a physician. A recommendation for admission by a physician was then followed by discussion and votes by the visiting committee of the Board of Trustees. Exceptions could be made, such as admission following a sudden accident or a patient who could afford to pay for their care. A board of managers provided the oversight of the hospital operations.

A number of people comprised the staff of the hospital and provided patient care. Foremost were the staff physicians who often served without pay, and they were assisted by medical students who served as interns. The physicians were assisted by a matron, a steward, and an apothecary, generally all paid positions. Stewards (also called Superintendents) and matrons were often husband and wife teams. Matrons bought supplies, kept hospital accounts, and hired and supervised other female employees (Tannenbaum 2012: 206). Stewards looked after enforcing rules of the hospital, and hired and fired personnel. Apothecaries saw to the purchase, preparation, and administration of medicine. Some had medical training, and they often worked with the physicians and medical students. Servants, coachmen, washerwomen, and attendants were also among the staff; most of the staff lived at the hospital (Rosenberg 1987: 38).

From the start, hospitals also served an educational function, that of clinical experience for physicians in training. The provision of clinical training at home in America was meant to stem the tide of medical students traveling to Europe (see Chapter 4). After sitting through two courses of lectures, medical students became eligible for their degree, but they received no clinical training in medical school. Hospitals provided "hands-on training," and newly minted doctors who had not received any clinical training were able to treat a variety of different conditions in hospital settings. The alliance of medical schools and hospitals thus fulfilled the needs of the community and served the additional function of keeping doctors in America for their training.

One function hospitals did not often serve during the first half of the nineteenth century was surgery or surgical training. Surgery was generally limited to setting fractures, righting dislocations, and treating ulcers and abscesses. Despite the introduction of ether in 1846, routine surgery was rare. "In October of 1858, for example, New York Hospital's First Surgical Division saw 109 patients treated but only 8 operations performed"

(Rosenberg 1987: 28). Because surgery was a last resort, and so few had an opportunity to practice it themselves, the surgical amphitheater became an important part of training physicians. The first surgical amphitheater in America was built in New York Hospital in 1803, with a second opening in Pennsylvania Hospital in 1804 (Duffy 1993).

General hospitals were plagued by problems despite the good intent of the philanthropic founders. It was clear by the end of the Revolutionary War that America's few general hospitals could not handle the growing number of worthy poor needing assistance. Overcrowded, and underfunded, hospitals were further implicated in the Jacksonian critique of professionalism (see Chapter 6). Adequate funding was always a problem, and tight funds led to inadequacies in all realms of hospital care and maintenance. The wards were overcrowded, and when surgeries were performed, they were all too often performed within the view of patients.

* * *

Numerous factors after 1750 conspired to instigate major changes in American social, political, and economic foundations. The collapse of the artisan system of labor separated the workplace from the home. Population growth, especially after 1800, swelled urban populations and the available number of laborers often exceeded the available work. People had trouble earning enough to live, and some turned to risky trades, some of which required extensive periods of time away from home. Housing and sanitation simply could not keep up with the increasing numbers of urban dwellers. Poverty became the normal family situation. Social and economic stratification, especially in New York, was accentuated as immigrants occupied crowded, unsanitary pockets of less-desirable neighborhoods, such as Five Points.

The erosion of family cohesion affected what health care was available and how it was implemented. Combined with poverty, America followed Britain in implementing support for the disfranchised and needy, first through outdoor relief and then with the establishment of institutional care. Those of sufficient economic means continued to practice most care within the home, but for many that was simply not possible. Establishing social care systems within the context of institutions was a new thing, and the growing pains were evident as it became apparent that life in those institutions was often unpleasant, unhealthy, and short. As medical professionalism emerged, America still had much to do about poverty and health care.

4

Licenses and Liabilities

Medical Training Becomes Formal

> From the mid-eighteenth century on, to be a physician or surgeon was to claim membership in an international healing cult whose character was scientific and anatomical.
>
> (Sappol 2002: 56)

> Medical men exert more influence on the manners of society, than any other class, except the rich.
>
> (Drake 1844: 20)

There was little impetus for a university-trained physician to emigrate to colonial America, and thus they were few and far between in the early colonies. Medicine in Europe during the sixteenth and the early seventeenth centuries was socially and professionally stratified and included several different kinds of practitioners. In seventeenth-century England, the highest-ranking were the physicians. They held medical degrees generally from Oxford or Cambridge and were members of the prestigious Royal College of Physicians (Duffy 1993: 7). Largely theoretical in nature, their training included only limited anatomical or clinical work. Physicians typically served their fellow upper-class citizens.

Surgeons and barber-surgeons were theoretically subject to physicians and were considered tradesmen. They dealt with physical tasks and treatments such as bloodletting, catheterizing, pulling teeth, dealing with injuries, and dressing wounds. Apothecaries compounded medicines and were also subject to physicians. Although neither surgeons nor apothecaries were university-trained, and thus not supposed to practice medicine, they were the practitioners accessible to the poorer classes. If individuals did have formal university education, they were frequently clergy, who formed a fourth medical specialization in America, the minister-physicians.

The social standing that university-trained physicians enjoyed in England was not immediately reinvented in colonial America, but it was eventually attained as both Soppol and Drake indicate above. Their membership in the upper class, and a clientele largely confined to that class, could not be duplicated in sixteenth- and seventeenth-century America. In fact, the social status that physicians held in England could hardly exist in the colonies, which were largely populated by the poorer segments of Britain and other parts of Europe. Most of the early settlers to the colonies were poor, often indentured servants, who could potentially enjoy better lives later after their servitude was completed. Consequently, until the mid- to late eighteenth century, American medical practitioners were largely trained through apprenticeships and formed the majority of the medical specialists.

Those who were trained through apprenticeship enjoyed higher status than they would have in Europe, and were able to practice medicine and refer to themselves as "doctors." The medical societies that supported regulation in Europe were slow to come to America, and regulation was minimal until the mid-eighteenth century. There was, in fact, little practical distinction between any of the types of healers in America until later.

Americans who wanted formal training in the seventeenth and early eighteenth centuries had to go to Europe to get it. Medical training was generally received at universities in Leiden, Edinburgh, and Glasgow. London hospitals offered training, but no formal degree. By the mid- to late eighteenth century, however, formal medical education became more prevalent both in Europe and America. Between 1749 and 1800, for instance, 103 American colonists attended the University of Edinburgh: 49 from Virginia, 16 from South Carolina, 15 from Pennsylvania, 10 from New York, 8 from Maryland, 3 from Georgia, and 2 from Massachusetts (Toledo-Pereyra 2006: 22).

Formally Trained Specialists

Medical Schools

Formal medical training in America began in New York in 1750 when physicians John Bard and Peter Middleton began offering private courses. Other private courses were offered in other cities. The first medical school in America was the Medical Department of the College of Philadelphia (later the University of Pennsylvania, 1766), and it was followed by King's College, New York (later Columbia University, 1767). Some would argue that earlier hospitals (for example, Charity Hospital in New Orleans) fulfilled the role of medical school, but they were more like almshouses (Duffy 1993: 35).

The Revolutionary War (1775–1783) slowed the growth of medical schools until 1810, although a few more were established. In 1782, a medical department was established at Harvard, and one in 1782 at Dartmouth. Transylvania University in Kentucky created a medical department in 1799, but medical courses were not given until 1817 and lasted only a short while; the department was closed by 1850 (Duffy 1993; Toledo-Pereyra 2006: 61–62).

After 1810, growth of medical schools accelerated in America, and by 1820, there were 20 medical schools in America, most located in New England. Coincident with the expansion of medical training in America between 1760 and 1860 was a growing number of physicians. Census figures for 1850 show that for every 100,000 people, there were 176 physicians, a number that surpassed both Britain and France (U.S. Department of Commerce 1: 76 [B 275–290] 1975). An additional 53 medical schools were founded by 1875. Interestingly, one of the last medical schools to open was Johns Hopkins in 1893.

Almost all schools were proprietary—they were supported by student funds. They were not connected to universities or hospitals, but were run independently by physicians who established the schools and who benefited both economically and socially through the prestige associated with them. It was a competitive business, and as the number of students and schools became more numerous, requirements became fewer; tuition fees formed the basic requirement (Devine 2014: 3). There were no standardized tests, college education, or literacy required.

Medical students generally attended two four-month terms of lectures, with the second offering the same content as the first. Admission to lectures was granted to anyone who could buy an admission ticket for about $20 from each professor whose class they attended (Duffy 1993: 134). The courses offered were fairly standard: anatomy, chemistry, botany, physiology, diseases of women and children, obstetrics, principles and practices of medicine and surgery (Devine 2014; Toledo-Pereyra 2006).

Clinical and hospital training were limited, but there was generally a one-to-three-year period of apprenticeship with a preceptor before graduating with a degree in medicine. In this regard, the apprenticeship system was still very much in place. In essence, the training of doctors had declined to simple lecture style training with very little "hands-on" experience, and even though they could obtain some further training as hospital interns, that experience was limited largely to care of chronic conditions. Surgery was hardly ever performed, and when it was, it generally involved fractures and ulcerative infections.

A Commerce of Dead Bodies

Anatomical training was handmaiden to the growth of the medical profession, and its transformation to a scientific profession. Anatomy and dissection were nothing new. After all, Vesalius had studied and presented his study of the human cadaver in *De humani corporis fabrica libri septem* in 1543. America between 1750 and 1870, however, was not prepared to recognize the importance of Vesalius' contributions, and thus, much of the impetus for anatomical training came from Europe.

Although thoroughly embraced in medical education, anatomical dissection was not embraced by the American general public. There were arguments to be made on both sides, religious and medical. The needs of the medical profession became more apparent as advances in surgery and an increasing number of surgical procedures necessitated knowledge of anatomy and skills in dissection. The need for cadavers, however, flew in the face of public sentiment and did little to endear medical school professors to the people.

Most physicians agreed that training in anatomy was fundamental to understanding the human body and its functions. The emphasis on anatomy and anatomical training was connected to a recasting of a physician's identity where surgery, once seen as a trade, became an essential part of medicine. Unfortunately, dead bodies on which to learn dissection were always in short supply and most were obtained by robbing graves. Public sentiment about the practice varied from place to place, but it was generally not viewed well.

Beliefs about the sanctity of the body in Anglo and American popular culture were not aligned with exhumation or dissection. In Christian thought, the body was sacred and had a significant role in providing a receptacle for the soul (Coffin 1976; Richardson 1987). Dead bodies were asleep for a period before the soul ascended to heaven; they were also powerful and dangerous to the living. There was a general sense that for a period following death, unspecified in length, the soul remained in the grave with the body; to exhume and dissect a corpse would prevent resurrection and ascension to heaven.

Compounding the liminal nature of the dead in the late eighteenth and nineteenth centuries, were oscillating waves of economic growth and collapse as America struggled to accommodate market capitalism; territorial expansion; dramatic urban growth; rapid technological advances in agriculture, industry, transportation, and communication; and substantial economic and social stratification. Tied to economic growth was a trend toward increased consumption—fashionable clothing and opulence in material goods spread far and deep, including into the aesthetics of death and mortuary ritual.

By the late eighteenth century, the funerary trade had firmly established normative standards—funerary urns and organized cemeteries with distinct plots ushered in the increased costs of death. Following the Civil War in Pittsburgh, a minimal working-class funeral cost between $75 and $100, close to $2,000 in today's currency (Kleinberg 1977). There was, nonetheless, the desire of the impoverished to bridge the chasm between the rich and poor, at least in the passage from life to death.

At the Uxbridge Almshouse burial ground in Massachusetts, a pauper's cemetery, archaeologists unexpectedly found that many coffins had decorative hardware. The poor, it turns out, did their best to signal a life lived, even while a lavish burial was out of financial reach, by adorning the caskets with mass-produced hardware that fell within their budget (Bell 1990).

Middle-class funeral expenses were far greater, an average of $500, close to $10,000 in today's economy, and the coffin hardware used in those mortuary treatments was handmade. Funerals and mortuary rituals allowed people to ritualize their identity against the tide of change; funerals became ostentatious affairs designed to authenticate one's social standing. Of course, this was all predicated on the assumption that one should stay in one's place of death permanently. In nineteenth-century America, many did not stay in their place of resting, and that somber fact troubled many Americans.

A number of variables governed whose bodies ended up on dissection tables and whose did not. Most medical schools required that there be no longer a period than ten days between death and exhumation; longer time periods made the amount of decay too difficult for dissection. Professional "body snatchers" or "resurrection men," as they were known, supplied medical schools with bodies for a standard fee of $5 to $25, depending on the age of the subject and the condition of the body (Duffy 1993: 132; McFarlin and Wineski 1997). Seasonality played a role in the magnitude of

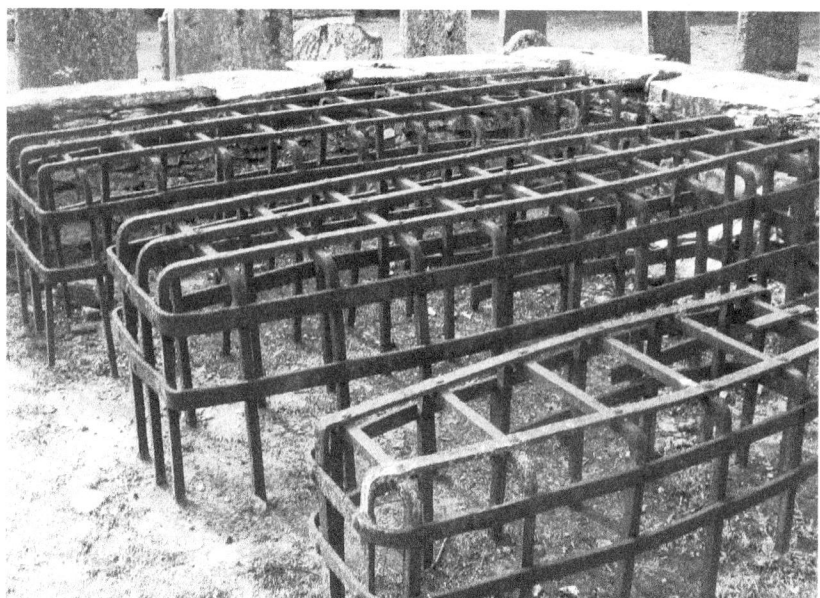

Figure 4.1. Mortsafes at a churchyard in Logierait, south of Pitlochry, Perthshire, Scotland. Photo by Judy Willson, https://commons.wikimedia.org/w/index.php?curid =5011645.

grave robbing—colder temperatures slowed decomposition and enabled longer distance transport.

The measures people took to protect the sanctity of their loved ones following death and burial were numerous. Families could hire guards for a short period or take turns watching over the grave of a loved one. The period of protection was limited given the short length of time that could pass before a body became unusable for dissection. Two of the simplest methods of protection were either to bury an individual near the residence or to have someone guard the grave for a period. Some families hired people to watch over the grave of their loved ones for a period of months following initial burial.

There were several alternative methods to face to face protection. A set of suspended bars known as a "mortsafe" had legs that went down into the ground and attached to the coffin (Figure 4.1.). A short-lived trend in coffin design was the iron coffin, which sometimes had windows. They were known as Fisk metallic burial cases, or Fisk Coffins after the inventor, Almond Fisk, and they were manufactured in Providence, Rhode Island. They had lids that were bolted down and sometimes even welded shut (Figure 4.2). Their popularity was limited to those of wealthier means; in the 1850s a pine coffin would have cost about $2 and a Fisk coffin about $100 (approximately $3,316 in today's currency). Their popularity was limited to the years from about 1850 until 1880.

With cemeteries located distant from the core of the population, the bodies of those with fewer financial resources—immigrants, paupers, and those of African descent—were differentially subjected to anatomical

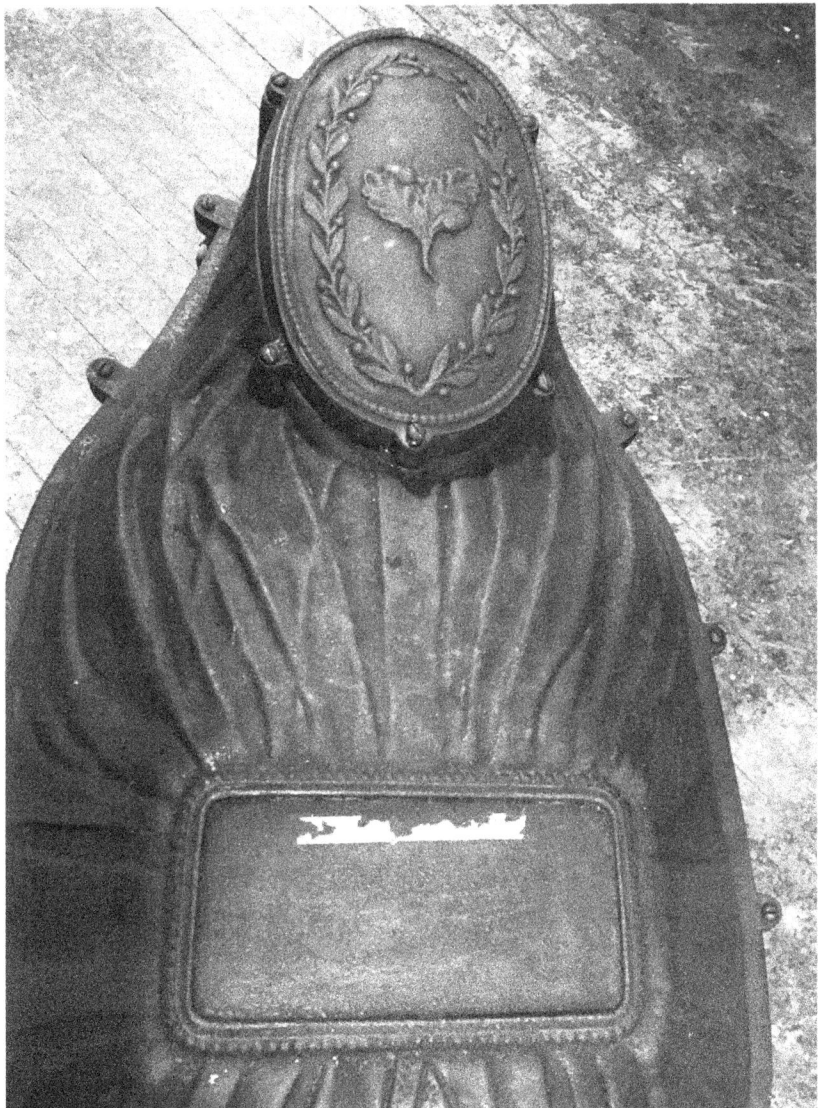

Figure 4.2. Fisk metallic burial case, circa 1850. The case is on display at the Canton Historical Museum in Collinsville, CT. Photograph credit: Scott Warnasch.

training. Burial grounds for African Americans were generally set away from busier parts of cities and were guarded less well. Dissection of Black cadavers throughout America was more common than that of Whites, as reported in the *Transylvania Medical Journal* (80 percent Blacks; Savitt 1982: 338) and in Baltimore (66 percent Blacks, Humphrey 1973: 824). The demand for cadavers was so great that grave robbers regularly shipped the corpses of southern Blacks to northern medical schools (Humphrey 1973), although Sappol (2002) reports that many cadavers were exported from New York as well.

Although the deterrents to grave robbing required time and money, there were methods available at lower cost in time and money to make the grave less penetrable, as reported in the late 1820s African-American newspaper, *Freedom's Journal*: "As soon as the corpse is deposited in the grave, let a truss of long wheaten straw be opened and distributed in layers, as equally as may be with every layer of earth, until the whole is filled up. By this method the corpse will be effectually secured; . . . the longest night will not afford time sufficient to empty the grave, though all the common implements of digging be used that purpose" (quoted in Sappol 2002: 14).

Dissection in medical education was thus viewed with disdain by the public, and the occasional flagrant act by medical students could inflame the issue. One such event resulted in the "doctor's riot" in New York. In 1788, a New York medical student dangled the arm of a cadaver out a window and told a passing boy that it was the arm of his mother. While undoubtedly concocted as a prank, the boy's mother had, in fact, recently died. Examination of her grave showed that the body was missing. A mob led by the boy's father rioted for two days, killing six people and destroying much of New York Hospital (Sappol 2002: 108). There were 20 such riots between 1785 and 1855, most targeted at medical schools, and a testament to public unrest over the use of cadavers (Sappol 2002).

The shortage of cadavers, combined with the public horror at grave robbing, led to two main responses. The first was to establish anatomy acts which would legally allow medical schools to dissect unclaimed bodies (Lusignan Lowe 2017; Sappol 2002). Those who were eligible for inclusion included felons, prisoners, the executed, and residents of almshouses. The logic underpinning decisions about who could be dissected ranged from a chance to serve society, having failed to do so during life, to punishment which presumably would act as a deterrent to bad behavior. The first such act was passed in Massachusetts in 1831, but it only pertained to Boston. A few other states joined in the passage of anatomy acts—Connecticut, New Hampshire, Michigan, New York—but by the Civil War only two states, Massachusetts and New York, had retained such legislation (Devine 2014: 3; Nystrom 2014).

The other response was for elite physicians to obtain anatomical training elsewhere. Anatomical training was conducted across eighteenth- and nineteenth-century Europe in places like Bologna, Leiden, Vienna, Paris, Edinburgh, and London. John and William Hunter were the primary figures teaching anatomy in London in the late 1700s, and their prestigious appointments—William as physician to Queen Charlotte and John as surgeon to King George III—gave plenty of sparkle to the Hunters' anatomy schools. American physicians who trained with the Hunters conveyed the message of the importance of anatomical training, but American public resistance remained.

Between 1830 and 1860, the Paris Clinical School was seen as the best and most advanced medical training facility in the world; elite American physicians found a refreshing change there from American medical training (Devine 2014; Rosenberg 1987). The Paris School made studying anatomy and participating in autopsies a fundamental part of understanding disease processes, a departure from the standard American passive bedside observation.

Students in Paris were able to compare lesions observed at the bedside with lesions observed postmortem through autopsy. Paris clinicians actively employed stethoscopes and other medical equipment novel to American medical students. Unfortunately, fewer than one thousand American physicians made the trip to Paris, and most physicians lacked much anatomical experience, at least legally (Devine 2014: 4). This is not to say that dissection was not practiced in America, quite the opposite. It was simply not the time for public acceptance of anatomical training, dissection, and the disfigurement of bodies in early- to mid-nineteenth-century America.

An Archaeology of Postmortem Disfiguration

Most American states had medical schools in the nineteenth century, and most emphasized the importance of anatomy, learned through dissection. Most had very little opportunity to acquire legal cadavers. That simple fact means that once those illegally obtained bodies had been dissected, they either had to be curated as specimens or clandestinely deposited somewhere. In states which had anatomy acts, the cadavers acquired often came from institutions which had their own burial grounds. One could assume that the remains from such institutions could be openly reburied in their burial grounds.

Burial in a cemetery still warrants an investigation as to the conditions and context of the burial. Whether in a coffin, casket, shroud, or simply in the earth, assessment of the way in which a person was buried might indicate something about their postmortem treatment. A "normal" burial should mirror the mortuary patterns of the time period and exhibit nothing out of the ordinary. Burials with multiple disarticulated elements, most exhibiting multiple cuts and saw marks not usually associated with autopsy, or that contain artifacts associated with display or teaching (for example, pins or hinges), or bones with a lot of fragmentation, do not signify normal burials.

It is important to distinguish between dissection and autopsy, and between medical experimentation and surgical amputation. Autopsy is a legitimate investigation into the cause of death, and because many of the almshouses were associated with hospitals, autopsies could account for some cases of postmortem modification (Dougherty and Sullivan 2017; Nystrom 2014: 770; Owsley et al. 2017). The amount of postmortem damage is usually less in autopsy cases.

Dissection, on the other hand, generally results in far more postmortem damage due to the number of people involved and the application of multiple procedures to multiple elements and element locations. Dissection was viewed in the eighteenth and nineteenth centuries as a violation; it "stripped the individual of their social identity and transformed the body into an object" (Nystrom 2011: 769). It was, in essence, structural violence in a way that autopsy was not. Autopsies were evidence that an individual was important enough to conduct an investigation into cause of death. Another important distinction is between surgical amputation and dissection. Surgical amputation should have a limited array of cuts, almost always performed with a saw, and may show evidence of healing.

Almshouses

There is a fair amount of archaeological and bioarchaeological evidence for the dissection of cadavers. Nystrom (2014) lists 24 archaeological sites exhibiting skeletal elements with postmortem damage. Much more detailed information for many of these sites is contained within the edited volume *The Bioarchaeology of Dissection and Autopsy in the United States* (Nystrom

2017). Several of these are the sites of almshouses, a frequent source of unclaimed bodies made available legally through the Anatomy Acts.

Of the eight almshouse sites Nystrom (2014) discusses, five have evidence of postmortem modifications, usually craniotomies (surgical opening of the skull). Most of them were located on very large properties away from the center of town to distance the indigent, sick, socially inept, and incarcerated away from the rest of the population. They commonly either had medical schools, hospitals, and other institutions on the property, or had close relationships with them. I focus below on three almshouse sites: the Albany County Almshouse, the Erie County Poorhouse, and the Blockley Almshouse.

The Albany County Almshouse opened in 1826 with 126 residents (Lusingnan Lowe 2017: 316). It was located on a 216-acre property known as Almshouse Square; also located there were a penitentiary, a pest house, and a cemetery. Adjacent to the property were the Albany Hospital and the Albany Medical School. From 1826 until 1926, Albany County Almshouse cemetery was the burial site for individuals at the almshouse, individuals from local hospitals and penitentiaries, and unclaimed bodies from the city of Albany (Nystrom 2014: 771).

Historical death records indicate that 312 bodies from the almshouse were claimed for dissection beginning in 1894 by the Albany Medical Center. Lusignan (2004: 771; Lusignan Lowe 2017) reported that 51 (5.7 percent) of the 903 individuals recovered from archaeological excavations at that cemetery exhibited cut marks that suggest they were dissected and used for surgical practice. Most were male (69 percent) and most showed evidence of craniotomies and/or transversely sectioned long bones. The small number of individuals recovered with evidence of dissection, as compared to the somewhat ambiguous historical records, suggests that most individuals were not placed back into mortuary contexts as normal burials.

Similar evidence of dissection was found at the Erie County Poorhouse, established in Buffalo in 1851. From the beginning, it served as the Erie County Hospital, an insane asylum, and a children's ward (Nystrom et al. 2017). It was associated with the Buffalo Medical Center. As a measure of service the facilities provided, during the 75 years it was in operation, 181,894 persons received care there. Before archaeological excavation of burials occurred in 2012, several road construction and campus improvement projects had identified 480 burial features (Nystrom 2014; Nystrom et al. 2017).

Eighty-seven of those features contained empty coffins; interestingly, an additional six had wood logs in them. Twenty individuals out of the MNI of 375 (5.3 percent) showed evidence of postmortem damage. Craniotomies were the most frequent type of damage, but there were also numerous transected long bones. While the latter could be the result of failed amputations, they have several additional cut marks that suggest more than simple amputation was practiced. As at the Albany County Almshouse, the Erie County Poorhouse males were more frequently the subjects of postmortem alterations (n=9, 45%) than were females (n=3, 15%) or juveniles (n=1, 5%).

Both of the almshouse examples discussed above come from individuals buried in graves as "normal" burials. The Anatomy Act for New York made it possible to legitimately provide burial for dissected individuals, although Nystrom (2014) suggests for the Albany County Almshouse that discrepancies between the number of burials exhibiting postmortem alterations and the written records imply that some dissected individuals did not get interred in the cemetery.

The Philadelphia Almshouse was first established in 1731 and occupied two locations near Independence Hall before declining property values led to moving it to a 187-acre property two miles away in Blockley County (Crist et al. 2017). It had an infirmary, renamed the Philadelphia Hospital in 1835, and also had connections with the University of Pennsylvania and Jefferson Medical College. The new institution could house 1,750 people, had an asylum for 400 children, and could treat 600 patients in the hospital. The Blockley Almshouse Cemetery was first used in 1865 (Crist et al. 2017). Students regularly interned at the almshouse hospital, where one can assume they did some combination of autopsy, dissection, and surgical intervention.

Archaeological excavations in 2001 confirm the assumption of postmortem treatment, but the patterns of burial differ from the New York almshouse sites. At Blockley, thousands of disarticulated skeletal elements were commingled and buried in 138 large boxes (1 ft. wide by 4 ft. long and 1 ft. deep) or simply dumped into pits. Some individuals were also interred in regular grave shafts. A demographic analysis using crania and mandibles showed that 67 percent of the 248 individuals were males, 30 percent were females, and 3 percent were indeterminate; no children were in the assemblage.

Biological anthropologists frequently make use of several methods to estimate sex and ancestry from the skeleton. Sex estimation is most frequently made by using visual assessment of morphological characters of the cranium, mandible, and pelvis, characters that are sexually dimorphic, for robusticity. Metric methods involve using discriminant function formulae or canonical correlate analysis to use established measurements that reflect sex and ancestry. These are most often applied to crania, mandibles, some long-bone diaphyses, and the head of the femur and humerus.

The measurements are initially taken from individuals of known sex in skeletal reference collections (for example, Terry collection at the Smithsonian or Hammond-Todd at the Cleveland Museum of Natural History). Because ancestry can exert considerable control on population robusticity, differences between males and females are usually assessed while also considering ancestry. The values of known sex and ancestry individuals yield weighting values which can be applied to skeletons for which those classifications are unknown.

Of Estimating Ancestry

Ancestry estimation similarly involves both visual methods of morphological character evaluation as well as mathematical discriminant function formulae. As with sex estimation, skeletal elements most conducive for ancestry estimation are the cranium and mandible. Ancestry was indeterminate for 71 percent of the 248 individuals from Blockley. Ancestry estimates of the crania and mandibles recovered from Blockley resulted in estimates that 24 percent were of European descent, 4 percent were of African descent, and 1 percent of Asian/Native American descent (Crist et al. 2017).

The discrepancies between historical records and the burials recovered archaeologically in New York raise questions about how many of those who underwent dissection or autopsy were returned to the ground. On the one hand, one could assume that the planned placement of the dead into an established space and place of death followed certain established societal norms that indicate a "normal" burial. On the other, though, mortuary spaces undergo repeated episodes of maintenance and disturbance, which could either clarify the conditions under which individuals were buried or it could distort them. One might get a somewhat less biased record if the actual site of the dissections is examined.

The Archaeology of Medical Schools and Dissection

Several medical school excavations provide the opportunity to see the disposal of the dead within the context of the training institution where the dissections were performed. The former building of the Medical College of Georgia is one of those institutions. Unlike New York, Georgia was one of the states that did not have an early anatomy act; until 1887, dissection of humans was illegal and was practiced without mention (Blakely 1997: 3). In Augusta, surgeons were trained in the dissection of human cadavers in a Greek Revival–style building constructed in 1835. It is likely cadavers, obtained through clandestine removal from graves, had to again be disposed of in a clandestine manner. They were probably not moved into public cemeteries.

In August of 1989, construction workers at the original building of the Medical College of Georgia (the medical school moved in 1912) discovered human bones in the earth floor of the basement. The materials recovered by the construction crew from the basement and areas adjacent to the building consisted of 9,808 human bones and bone fragments, about 300 animal bones, and nearly 2,000 artifacts (Blakely 1997). Given the elements recovered, the minimum number of individuals is estimated to be 62, although Blakely and Harrington suspect the actual number of individuals buried at the college to be somewhere between 200 and 400 (Blakely 1997: 11). Most of the artifacts date to the 1800s, and in combination with the animal and human bones, provide a window into a rather secretive part of surgical training during that period.

Of the 9,808 human skeletal elements and bone fragments, 389 (4 percent) show signs of postmortem cuts attributed to dissection and/or amputation (McFarlin and Wineski 1997). There undoubtedly would have been saws employed in the amputations and dissections, but none were mentioned in the list of artifacts (Blakely and Harrington 1997). Two thirds of those bones showing cuts are on postcranial elements (n=279), while 110 are on cranial bones. Almost all of the postcranial bones exhibiting cuts were severed completely.

Blakely and Harrington used metric analysis of the tibiae to estimate the ancestry of the dissected elements. The tibia has fairly robust accuracy for ancestry estimation (70.5 percent for females and 82.9 percent for males; Krogman and İşcan 1986: 290–91). Their discriminant function estimates for the 24 tibiae they could examine showed that most individuals (n=19; 79%) were of African descent (Harrington 1997: 277). A chi-square test showed the difference in number of African Americans to Euro-Americans (n=5) to be significant at the $p<.001$ level (Blakely and Harrington 1997: 174).

A number of artifacts were recovered from the Medical College of Georgia excavations. There were bottles, many of which contained alcohol, medicines, or other chemicals. There were utilitarian ceramic jugs and vessels. One packing bottle with a glass stopper contained human fetal lung tissue that was immersed in whiskey as a preservative (Duncan 1997). Medical and laboratory artifacts included scalpels, pipettes, syringes, test tubes, thermometers, and microscope slides. A latrine in one corner contained dissected skeletal remains, as did a large wooden vat that historical records mention was used to preserve cadavers and body parts (Allen 1976).

The Medical College of Virginia at Virginia Commonwealth University was established in 1854, although from 1838 it was formerly part of the Medical Department of Hampton-Sydney College. The Egyptian Building, which opened up in 1844, included an infirmary, patient beds, a dissecting room, and lecture rooms. The site became the subject of archaeological investigations when a construction crew discovered a circular brick well that contained animal bones, human bones, building debris, personal items, and medical implements (Owsley et al. 2017). Among the medical items were glass test tubes, pharmaceutical bottles, a thermometer, bone scalpel handles, and ointment pots.

Anatomy was always an important part of the college training in Richmond, and so the discovery of human bones was not surprising. Like Georgia, Virginia had no anatomy act and so cadavers had to be supplied by resurrection men, although it is highly likely that some cadavers came from those who died in the infirmary. Study of the human skeletal remains revealed that there were a minimum of 44 adults and 9 children (Owsley et al. 2017).

There were 26 partial and complete crania for which sex estimates were made: 17 (65 percent) were male, 8 were female (31 percent), and 1 was indeterminate. The majority of the crania (n=18; 69%) were of African ancestry, as discerned through metric estimates, while only 2 (8%) were of European descent. Ancestry estimates were not possible for the remaining 6. Thirty-five of the crania and mandibles of the 196 present exhibited "intentional sectioning consistent with dissection and surgical training in surgical procedures including amputations and autopsy (Owsley et al. 2017: 151). Forty-two postcranial elements of the total number of 558 show evidence of dissection (see Owsley et al. 2017: Figure 4.2). One adult scapula had a metal hook in the glenoid fossa (see Owsley et al. 2017: Figure 4.3) which was used to attach to the humerus for anatomical display.

Holden Chapel at Harvard University, as the name suggests, was originally designated as a place of worship when built in 1744, but it was retrofitted in 1801 to house the Harvard Medical School (Hodge et al. 2017). Human and animal bones, as well as personal items and those involved in medical training, were recovered from a well in 1999. Among the artifacts were a bowl, a chamber pot, beer bottles, an inkwell, buttons, and shoes. Most of the artifacts pertained to nineteenth-century anatomical training and included test tubes, graduated cylinders, slides, flasks, specimen jars, and crucibles. They were contained in several layers and provide bracketed dates of roughly 1785–1860 (Hodge et al. 2017: 120). There were 2,748 animal-bone fragments and 907 human skeletal elements representing 16 individuals. No intact skeletons were found.

Of the 907 human bones, 757 were adult and 38 came from juveniles. From these skeletal elements, the investigators estimate an MNI of 12 adults and 4 juveniles. Sex estimates were only possible for five individuals; unlike the prior two medical school examples, males and females were more or less equally represented. Cut marks were observed on 51 cranial and postcranial elements that are consistent with dissection. No estimates of ancestry were made by the authors. As in other states, medical acts came slowly and so prior to 1831 " . . . the dissection of anyone besides executed criminals and suicides was illegal in Massachusetts" (Hodge et al. 2017: 132). However, a series of anatomy acts passed in Massachusetts in 1831, 1834, and 1845 increased the availability of cadavers.

These archaeological case studies demonstrate that anatomical training was widespread in America in the eighteenth century. In the eyes of medical professionals, it legitimated the profession and ushered in an increased awareness of anatomy and surgical intervention. Dissection of cadavers was not limited simply to medical school, and was likely practiced during other periods of a medical professional's life. Archaeological testing in 1985 in Annapolis, Maryland, revealed evidence of such anatomical experimentation at the site of a practicing physician, Dr. Frank Thompson (Mann et al. 1991).

In a privy at the site, two partial femora were recovered, a right and left, which are probably from the same individual. The left femur has surgical cuts on both the proximal and distal ends, but performed with different techniques and instruments. The right femur was surgically altered in exactly the same way as the left. One of the authors of the article has examined hundreds of skeletal elements from amputations of Civil War soldiers, and they do not match the techniques or locations of the cuts on the bones found in the privy; they likely were postmortem anatomical experimentation.

* * *

The chasm between physicians and the public widened in the early to mid-nineteenth century. Public distrust of anatomical training was no small contributor to that distrust.

5

Suspect Specialists

> The planter, the farmer, the mechanic, and the laborer all know that their success depends upon their own industry and economy, and that they must not expect to become suddenly rich by the fruits of their toil. Yet these classes of society form the great body of the people of the United States; they are the bone and sinew of the country.... The mischief springs from the power which the moneyed interest derives from a paper currency which they are able to control, from the multitude of corporations with exclusive privileges which they have succeeded in obtaining in the different States, and which are employed altogether for their benefit.
>
> (Andrew Jackson, Farewell Address, March 4, 1837)

Andrew Jackson, the seventh president of the United States between 1829 and 1837, is best known for three things. One was his desire to preserve the Union, which was under assaults from numerous corners. The second was his signing of the Indian Removal Act in 1830, a piece of legislation that resulted in the relocation of hundreds of thousands of Native Americans from their homeland. A third was his advocacy for the common laborer against the corrupt aristocratic wealthy and elite.

It was in this context that the American medical system, if it could be called that, foundered in the early to mid-1800s. Physicians did little to help themselves until about 1850, decades after the emergence of several popular, alternative movements in health and well-being. Fueled by the Jacksonian "anyone can be a professional" movement, physicians became suspect specialists.

Physicians and Medical Schools

By the early nineteenth century, tensions about the scientific professionalism in medicine stretched widely across public sentiment. There were also aspects of physician training that were not fully accepted. As more and more medical schools opened, qualifications were virtually reduced to having the available funds to pay for the tickets for training. The elimination of entrance requirements in proprietary medical schools, and the very short two sessions of four months with little clinical training (although internships were frequently required), meant that a rising tide of poorly trained licensed physicians flooded the populace. After about 1820, concerns about the slack approach to physician training began to emerge.

Anatomical dissection was another area of concern for many people. With the increase in medical schools, the need for cadavers increased while the supply remained low. Body snatching had done nothing to create a favorable impression of medical training and practice. The elitism of licensed medical professionals amid an untrusting public acted against their best interest. Hospitals were commonplace, but they were struggling to be financially solvent, as well as to be healthy places to receive treatment and convalesce. In fact, there was growing sentiment that institutional health care was not a great approach.

Laws benefiting university-trained physicians were another source of professional tension. In 1736, Virginia passed a law specifying charges for standard fees and mileage for out-of-town visits. It also allowed university-trained physicians to charge twice as much as apprentice-trained doctors, and both New York and New Jersey attempted to enact licensing laws. The development of professional organizations, known as medical societies, in the mid-eighteenth century was a sure sign of an emerging professionalism.

Between 1750 and 1790, medical societies were established in Boston, Charleston, Connecticut, Massachusetts, and New Jersey. They generally served to legitimate formally trained physicians, and to formally rebuke "quacks, mountebanks, imposters, or other pretenders of medicine" (Duffy 1993: 42), while ensuring larger fees for services. They were frequently criticized for attempting to create a professional monopoly.

Public distrust was also directed at the methods of treatment practiced by many formally trained physicians. From about 1780 until 1830, most physicians were engaged in "heroic medicine." Following the belief that health and wellness were controlled by bodily humours, heroic physicians practiced active intervention in the course of a sickness. A strong supporter of heroic medicine, and perhaps one of the most well-reputed colonial physicians, was Benjamin Rush, a signer of the Declaration of Independence who was associated with the Philadelphia Medical Hospital.

The active interventions that Rush and other heroic doctors favored were accomplished by bloodletting, purging, and sweating to shock the body into returning to humoural balance. Physicians frequently resorted

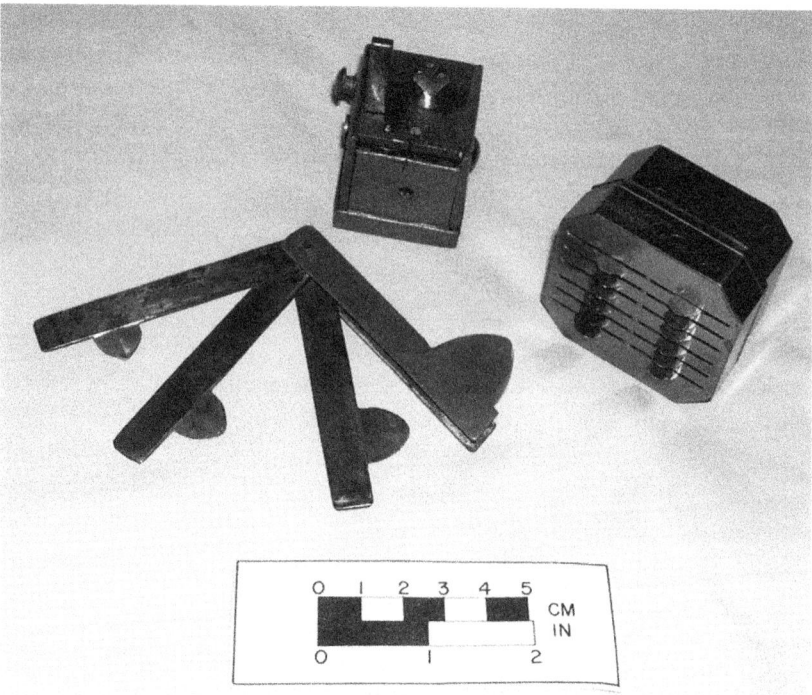

Figure 5.1. Scarificators (*top and right*) and lancets (*bottom left*). Photographed by the author at the Country Doctor Museum, Bailey, NC.

to bleeding using lancets and scarificators for opening up blood vessels (Figure 5.1). Lancets generally had one or two blades, much like a jackknife, which folded out and could be used to penetrate the skin. Scarificators were more sophisticated and had four to sixteen blades recessed in a casing. When released, the composite set of blades was released, causing ample bleeding. Heated glass cups were placed above the openings made by lancets and scarificators, and these created suction that drew infection from open wounds. Leeches were also often used to draw blood; any good physician's office or apothecary had them in stock, often in elaborately decorated ceramic jars.

Blistering was accomplished by placing mustard plasters of Spanish fly (Cantharides, derived from beetles) or some other substance on the skin to cause a second-degree burn (Duffy 1993: 71). It was thought those treatments released bad humours. Calomel, a white powdered form of mercuric chloride, was the most common drug prescribed and was administered to cause purging, either through diarrhea or vomiting. Other frequently prescribed drugs were opium, ipecac, and camphor, the latter two often combined with opium.

George Washington's treatment in 1799 serves to illustrate a standard course (Duffy 1993: 73–74). Washington was suffering from an acute throat infection, and he was initially bled and his throat blistered with Cantharides, while leeches were placed on his throat and behind his ears. When those procedures did not work he was administered an enema, given several more doses of calomel and tartar, and bled twice more. As he grew increasingly frail, two more physicians entered the scene and removed another 32 ounces of blood, now coming thick and slow. Washington died that night.

The increase in formally trained physicians had a number of impacts on a youthful America. For one, it eventually reinforced the emerging social stratification of the colonies, not only because of the social status of doctors, but because of the choices that the upper classes made to engage their services. Furthermore, despite the popularity of formally trained physicians by the upper class, lay practitioners and those trained through apprenticeships continued to be those professionals more accessible to the less wealthy. It seemed clear about 1830 that public distrust of physicians, especially heroic physicians, would necessitate changes in the system.

Revisionist Movements and the Common Person

Alongside public disdain for the study of human cadavers, there was a marked turn away from professional authority after 1820, especially from those formally trained as medical specialists. The attacks on medical professionalism arose not out of a vacuum, but as a larger social response during a time of independent thought in American culture. Distrust of professionals was not limited to physicians, but was part of a growing movement in the early nineteenth century that stressed "anyone can be a professional." Certainly the divisions within the field of medicine between those licensed and formally trained, and those not, did not strengthen the public image of physicians.

The movement was particularly fueled by President Andrew Jackson. Jackson promoted a spirit of egalitarianism with a distrust of intellectuals and learning, and his "Jacksonianism" considered privileged elites as parasites on the general good of America. Coincident with a growing public disdain for university-trained medical specialists in the 1820s and 1830s was public skepticism of some of the central practices of heroic doctors.

Bloodletting, and the administration of mercurials, arsenics, and other dangerous drugs, fell under intense criticism.

Another response of the Jacksonian movement was to reemphasize the role of spirituality in health. In essence, morality and health went hand in hand as religious revivals swept across America prior to the Civil War. There were increasing numbers of people advocating a less harsh, less directly interventive approach to medicine, and a number of alternative medical approaches, one might say schools of thought, emerged after 1800. Many were named for the innovator of the approach. Among those who saw themselves more as "interpreters of science" were William Alcott, Sylvester Graham, James C. Jackson, and Mary Gove; all are names often seen as lay health reformers (Green 1986).

Health reformers in the 1830s and 1840s were of various types—physical fitness advocates, water-cure specialists, electromagnetizers, dietary reformers—but they all shared a distrust of and opposition to the established medical profession. They offered individual Americans the opportunity to take their personal health care into their own hands, assisted at times by lay practitioners. Most health revisionist movements stressed the importance of organic treatments over the use of drugs, although patent medicines did find their way into some treatment plans.

One person who sat between reformers and professionals was Edward Hitchcock, a professor of geology and natural sciences at Amherst College. He was a well-known paleontologist who had made several important finds, and he was also the third president of Amherst College. While Hitchcock was certainly not always admired by health reformers, he did advocate a healthy diet, and he was the first physical education professor in America (Green 1986: 12). In 1830, Hitchcock put many disease symptoms under the term "dyspepsy or dyspepsia" (Hitchcock 1831). The symptoms, or diseases, ranged from those that included mental conditions to various digestive disorders.

Another very influential character was Samuel Thomson, who referred to educated physicians as "educated quacks" and under whose tutelage sprang a domestic health movement known as the "Thomsonians." His book, *Learned Quackery Exposed,* was written in verse:

> Let the names of all disorders be,
> Like to the limbs joined on a tree;
> Work on the root, and that will subdue,
> Then all the limbs will bow to you;

So as the body is the tree,
The limbs are cholic, pleurisy,
Worms and gravel, gout and stone
Remove the cause and they are gone.
My system's founded on this truth,
Man's Air and Water, Fire and Earth,
And Death is cold, and life is heat,
These temper'd well, your health's complete. (Thomson 1824: 22)

Samuel Thomson was an advocate of purging through vegetative compounds and sweating, which he maintained would "unclog the bodily system." Shunning professional medical care of the time in the form of bleeding, blistering, purging, and tonics, Thomson chose to emphasize healing based on herbs and steam—less severe methods of healing (Thomson 1822). He did not favor formal medical education but rather empirical observation. Thomson's appeal to commoners of the rural South and Midwest was his written presentation in plain English and his fervent denouncement of formal medical education.

His reactionary stance and public appeal were fueled by the Jacksonian movement. Any Jacksonian American ought to not only be able to choose their own physician, but they should be able to practice as one if they wanted to do so. Thomson and other health reformers aimed to end what they saw as a legal monopoly on practicing medicine by targeting medical licensing laws. It was extremely successful and in the 1840s all but three states ended licensing laws (Armstrong and Armstrong 1991: 27).

Thomson created a system of medicine, and his six courses of treatments combined vomiting, often brought about by lobelia (*Lobelia inflata*, commonly known as Indian tobacco or puke weed); scalding herbal teas; enemas; infusions; and steam vapor (Armstrong and Armstrong 1991: 25). Thomson's appeal was cross-cultural. It presented a natural means for self-health that avoided the harsh treatments prescribed by doctors, such as calomel, which contained mercury. Thomsonian medicines were carried on the Trail of Tears by the Cherokee (Armstrong and Armstrong 1991: 26). In fact, Thomsonian favorites such as lobelia and steam baths had long been used in Native America.

Thomson sold "family right certificates" for $20, which yielded a 20-page booklet and membership in "Friendly Botanic Societies." Most of his sales were conducted by agents who sold the memberships as well as his branded "American Made" medications. Between 1811 and 1839, Thompson claims that he made $2 million from his sales of 100,000 certificates and medications (Duffy 1993: 81–82). That figure is $55,508,602 in today's currency.

Homeopathic medicine was another revisionist movement. It originated in Germany about 1800 and is often associated with Samuel Hahnemann (Armstrong and Armstrong 1991; Green 1986). The premise of homeopathy is that a sick person can be cured by giving them small doses of some natural compound that causes similar symptoms. It is an approach, while often attributed to Hahnemann's systematic investigations, that was also practiced among Native Americans. Constantine Hering is the person in America most closely noted for practicing homeopathic medicine, and who founded the Hahnemann Medical School in Philadelphia.

Sylvester Graham, in many ways, epitomized the popularized turn away from specialist professionalism. Graham was a dynamic preacher, well known for his arguments that regular exercise, fresh air, vegetarian diet, temperance with regard to alcohol, and regular bathing were the keys to a healthy life. Remembered mostly today for his dedication to "you are what you eat," the cracker that bears his name and is found on grocery shelves today hardly resembles the coarse whole-grain bread he advocated. Graham successfully reached thousands of health-conscious Americans, who were known as Grahamites.

So widespread was Graham's notion of meatless meals that if someone were a vegetarian, it was assumed they were a Graham follower. In addition to his dietary regimen, his recommendation for loose, comfortable clothing was well received by women in the age of corsets. Long after his death in 1851, his followers continued to forward his message of fresh air, water cures, vegetarianism, exercise, and temperance, among them William Alcott, Catherine Beecher, and John Harvey Kellogg.

Physicians Fail Legitimacy

Amid the rising tide of voices in alternative health-care movements, most speaking out against "allopathic" medicine (science-based medicine), university-trained physicians were forced to respond. The responses were generally at the state level, although a national effort was made in 1846 to shore up training at the first meeting of the National Medical Convention (later to become the AMA). The committee that was assigned at the meeting to make recommendations had several: (1) increase the academic year to two six-month terms, (2) demand proof of internship, and (3) ensure that each school have at least seven faculty (some schools had as few as three), each specializing in one of the seven major topics (medicine, surgery, anatomy, physiology and pathology, pharmacy, midwifery and gynecology, chemistry and medical law)(Duffy 1993). Those schools that adopted the new standards, among them the University of Pennsylvania and the College of Physicians and Surgeons in New York, soon found that students attended other schools with lower standards.

The American Medical Association (AMA) was founded in 1847. The AMA promoted education through its journal, the *Journal of the American Medical Association* (JAMA), and attempted to provide a central unifying organization for the medical profession. Unification, however, faced many obstacles. Even the medical schools participated in the licensing debate. They asserted that the qualifications of a physician were matters for the institution; once they had recognized that the training and internships of a student were complete, it was their role to grant the degree, and therefore the license.

There were other criticisms beyond professional training, however. Licensing was a target of many critics. Those who lacked formal education saw licensing as "gatekeeping." The various alternative health movements saw licensing as the creating of monopolies. Many states, however, disagreed and insisted that they held the primary role of licensing.

Given all of the criticisms of formally trained physicians, it seemed to many people that doctors were paid an awful lot of money. The income of physicians, many of whom practiced in urban environments, was substantial. Their services, ranging from teaching to consultations with patients, could yield salaries of around $10,000 if they had attended a good medical school, with part of their training in Europe (Duffy 1993). If we assume a date of 1830 for that salary, it was $280,600 in contemporary monetary value.

Many physicians did not make that kind of salary, as they practiced in smaller towns or rural environments. Country doctors saw people on their own premises. However, during disease epidemics and seasonal diseases (for example, measles), they made house calls and were often out healing people most evenings. Dr. William Lay Smith of Hertford County charged his patients by the number of miles he traveled plus a set charge for his services. Between 1806 and 1810, he charged 50 cents for a puke or purge, a dollar for a tooth extraction, and 40 cents per mile of travel. Another example is Dr. Goforth of Cincinnati, the physician to whom Daniel Drake was apprenticed. Drake reported that typical charges for people in that rural environment were 25 cents for bleeding, 25–50 cents for a visit, one dollar for sitting up all night with them, and 25 cents per mile for travel (Duffy 1993: 141).

Those salaries were certainly far from $10,000 per annum, and many country doctors owned farms and other enterprises to supplement their income. Often as not, payment to country doctors was accepted in vegetables, fruits, meat, and labor. The literature on country doctors is scant and mostly consists of journals and small references (for example, Hubbard 1998; Parramore 1971). There is a wonderful Country Doctor Museum in Bailey, North Carolina, and they maintained a digital website where one can view many of the artifacts on display.

Despite its appeal to many in the rural South and Midwest, the Jacksonian-influenced movement against medical professionals may well have been differentially endorsed and more prevalent in urban environments. Country doctors seem to have remained in favor during the nineteenth and early twentieth centuries, perhaps due to the "down to earth" mannerisms and their dedication to doctoring. They were often highly respected members of the community who engaged across social, political, gender, and racial lines.

It did not escape the attention of the public that within the professional physician's community there was considerable discord. Some of it existed because of the social and professional stratification that resulted from training and from location of practice. Disagreements among physicians about the causes of various ailments certainly fueled public distrust. Between about 1820 and 1870, the actual causes of disease were hotly debated. Some, like Dr. Daniel Drake, put great emphasis on meteorological conditions, soil, topography. Drake spent a lot of time attending to those afflicted by malaria and yellow fever, and his treatise on those diseases (Drake 1850: 727) emphasized the formation of diseases in place given the right conditions.

> People who inhabit houses built on the hills adjoining valleys, are said to suffer more than those who reside below. Now every breeze may waft and lodge in such habitations the microscopic beings which multiply in the rich and humid valley-soil. It has also been observed, that a grove of forest trees between an uninhabited house, and what is called a sickly spot, gives comparative immunity from the Fever; and may not the leaves of such trees as successfully arrest animulcules,

or vegetable germs, as they can absorb a gas not designed for their nourishment? (Drake 1850: 727)

Others embraced theories of diseases being brought into localities, although the mechanisms were not really understood.

There were numerous permutations regarding the origin and cause of disease, which resulted in bitter disputes, rivalries, and even several duels (Duffy 1993: 144–145). Combined with debates among and between medical societies about licensing and who controlled it, medical schools or state governments, and a growing distrust of the public, there was little solidarity that could be brought to bear. In addition, the growing number of practicing physicians led to competition and charges of stealing patients.

By the mid-nineteenth century, the care that was associated with hospitals had come heavily into question. Studies in Britain, France, and America all pointed to the dangers of hospital-originated fevers and infections that made treatment in a hospital more dangerous than care at home, and thus the term "hospitalism" emerged (Rosenberg 1987: 122). Hospitalism referred to the increased danger of medical care in a hospital, as compared to home health care, and the issue was on the minds of many. Furthermore, the risk of hospital-borne infections increased coincident with increases in the size of the hospital. As the evidence of a problem became more widely apparent, there were numerous calls for reform.

Physicians as Suspicious Innovators

The period between 1830 and 1860 was marked by increasing distrust of heroic medicine and the harsh treatments associated with it. However, the numerous medical innovations and practices that emerged during that time were not fully embraced either. New instruments, such as the stethoscope and thermometer, offered new diagnostic resolution, but had little initial impact on American medicine of the time; anesthesia and antiseptics, also novel, were not widely applied. Archaeological investigations in New Brunswick, New Jersey, offer material evidence of medical practices less apparent in historic records.

Block 44 of New Brunswick was the subject of excavations conducted in late 1986 and early 1987 (Veit 1996). Two doctors practiced medicine on the property. The first was Dr. Clifford Morrogh who arrived there in 1847 with a newly minted MD from the City University of New York. Morrogh was a skilled surgeon who performed several notable surgical treatments, and was one of the first physicians in the United States to make use of anesthesia using chloroform. His office and residence were constructed in 1851 on Albany Street and were his main site of medical operations until his death of a heart attack on March 13, 1882. He was succeeded by his assistant, Dr. Donahue, who purchased the property in 1890.

Feature One was a rectangular stone-lined foundation, probably the location of a one-story structure shown on insurance maps. Over 200 medical and hygiene-related artifacts were recovered from Feature One, and included test tubes, syringes, eye droppers, beakers, a crucible, graduated cylinders, scalpels, and 97 pharmaceutical bottles (Veit 1996). Unfortunately, chronological assignments for the artifacts are difficult given the fact that an episode of construction and one of pot hunting commingled materials, and we must simply treat them as discards between 1851 and 1919, the year of Dr. Donahue's death. It was also impossible to determine whether they had resulted from one or multiple deposits.

The artifact assemblage is important because it expands the perception of physicians' roles and practices at the time. Historical records highlight the role of the two physicians with regard to surgery, but the archaeological assemblage reveals that their practices were far more diverse. The artifacts serve to illustrate the numerous roles, some unexpected, which physicians fulfilled and which might have been upsetting to some citizens.

Instruments and vessels found at the site went beyond those employed in surgery, to those used for diagnosis, those used for preparation of medicines, and those used for anesthesia and for gynecology. Several of these medical applications were likely to have been viewed with suspicion. Among the implements recovered from the excavations of Dr. Morrogh's Well, many relate to women's health, among them several hard-rubber pessaries and a vaginal syringe (Figure 5.2). Pessaries were used to relieve discomfort and reposition a prolapsed uterus, as well as to prevent miscarriages. They became popular in the 1860s after Hugh Lenox Hodge (Hodge 1866: 416–417) modified the centuries-old devices by manufacturing them out of vulcanized rubber.

There were also fifteen other fragmentary large syringes recovered which might also be vaginal syringes. Cleansing the vagina with bulb syringes (douching) became a prevalent form of birth control after 1930. The large number of gynecological implements found indicates that the physicians were actively treating women. The involvement of professional physicians in the mid-nineteenth century in gynecology would have been novel; James Marion Sims of Montgomery, Alabama, was the first doctor in the United States to provide gynecological surgery in 1845 (see discussion below). The

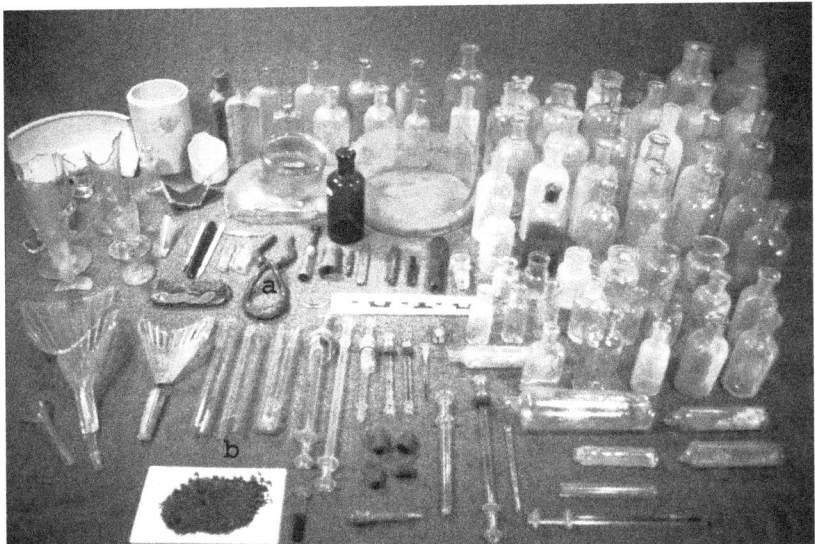

Figure 5.2. Items from Feature One, Dr. Morrogh's Well, including, in clockwise order: pharmaceutical bottles; ointment pots; graduated cylinders; funnels; a soil sample; and syringes. Located in the center-left portion of the photograph are pessaries (*a*), and vaginal syringes (*b*). Originally published in *Northeast Historical Archaeology* (1996, Richard Veit, Fig. 4). Permission to reprint provided by *Northeast Historical Archaeology*; photograph provided by Richard Veit.

majority of attention to women's reproductive health had been under the auspices of midwives until that point.

Another innovation revealed by the Block 44 excavations was anesthesia, hardly known in the mid-nineteenth century. Ether was used first in 1846 for a dental extraction in Boston, and was followed in 1847 by the discovery of chloroform by Dr. James Simpson working in Edinburgh. Dr. Morrogh was one of the first American surgeons to perform surgery using chloroform in 1847. He and Dr. Augustus F. Taylor amputated the leg of two injured African-American men from the local poorhouse using chloroform.

However, the use of anesthetics was accepted only slowly. Some viewed the interruption of pain as a hindrance to the healing process. Some voiced concerns about "moral dangers" to women who were anaesthetized. Those adhering to heroic medicine saw it as a sharp departure from the bleeding and aggressive treatments they provided. It took the Civil War (see Chapter 6) to bring about general acceptance of anesthesia, a transition which took place in no small part under the guidance of Dr. James Morrogh. Some of the smaller syringes at the site may indicate the injection of anesthetics, a practice for morphine injection widely used in the Civil War.

There are potentially some darker sides to the gynecological treatment of women. Dr. J. Marion Sims is credited with development of the first consistently successful operation for curing vesicovaginal fistula, a complication of childbirth where a hole develops between a woman's bladder and vagina. The resulting incontinence is unremitting. However, the charges against Sims are disturbing. He treated numerous women of African descent who were enslaved, and whose permission has been questioned. Some of those women experienced numerous operations. He is charged with performing those vaginal surgeries without administering anesthesia, which was available at the time, although not so widely accepted, and yet he apparently performed gynecological surgery on women of European descent with anesthesia (NPR 2018). There is debate on Sims's ethics, and there are those who challenge his violation of those ethics (for example, Wall 2006). Nonetheless, Sims's actions prompted the removal of his statue from Central Park in New York.

* * *

By the eve of the Civil War in 1861, the roles and practices of physicians in America were challenged from a number of fronts. Anatomical training in most states was not legally possible. Public sentiment about the elitist medical specialists had fostered numerous alternative specialist roles. Disagreements among physicians regarding the origins of diseases and treatment plans further undermined public support. The medical needs of a country torn by war within its own borders, however, would soon turn attention to the very real needs of health and well-being within.

III

Reformation and Reconstruction, 1850–1900

6

The Civil War and the Reformation of American Medicine

> War seems to be a social necessity. It is in human nature. It has existed ever since the beginning of Creation and will probably continue to exist as long as there are men,—consequently passions, errors and prejudices.—In spite of all the reasoning of philosophers and moralists, in spite of all the efforts of the Peace League to suppress it, war will occur, and Universal Peace remain an utopia. The sword will always be of a mighty weight in the balance of the destiny of nations.
>
> (Formento 1863: 4)

War (armed conflict) brought misery and mortality back to back. Misery, in the form of famine, festering wounds, disease, and dysentery, often met mortality not in the front lines, but in the camps or many months later. Yet, this knowledge, as Formento states, has not stifled the necessity of war. Like modern wars, mortality in the past was sometimes immediate, but in the wars before the nineteenth century, weapons often did not have the strength or accuracy to kill immediately. Rather, they permanently altered physical (bodily) structures or created the wounds that opened a person up to infection. Survival, if it was to occur, was often at the expense of severe disfigurement and lessened physical abilities. War was, and still is, not a pretty picture.

There have been many wars in many countries that have seen the involvement of American troops, but none has reflected purely American issues or changed the face of American medicine more than the Civil War. Known also as the War Between the States, the War of the Rebellion, and here in my adopted Southern homeland, as the War of Northern Aggression, it was a purely American conflict. It was fought by Americans, against each other, over an issue not purely American—slavery.

The Civil War and Medical Reformation

It seems ironic that the Civil War should bring about reformation in the American medical system, but it did just that. In 1861, the year the first battles of the Civil War occurred, the hygienic condition of hospitals was abysmal, and fears of hospitalism abounded. The period between 1830 and 1860 thus was one not only of stagnation for the medical profession, but of retrenchment (see Chapters 4 and 5). Social movements against elitism, medical school training, medical legislation, and a number of other things left physicians relatively unregulated and inexperienced. There was widespread debate about the importance of hygiene, what caused contagion, and the origin of disease agents.

It was in this context that the Civil War broke out in 1861, and the dramatic scale and immediacy of wound treatment, amputation, and sterilization found American military medical personnel totally unprepared (Adams 1996; Cunningham 1958; Gross 1862; Kuz and Bengtson 1996). The scale of sickness in military camps and the destructiveness of battle wounds surpassed anything previously seen in the American medical profession. The two major causes of death (other than trauma) were posttrauma infections and diseases of hygiene such as diarrhea and dysentery. By the time the Civil War ended in 1865, it had claimed between 600,000 and 750,000 lives from battle wounds, disease, or accidents (Duffy 1993; Hacker 2011).

The mortality figures hardly capture the grave extent of the impacts on the soldiers' health, however. Far more deaths were caused by sickness than wounds, a ratio of approximately 3:1 for Confederate forces and 2:1 for those from the Union (Duffy 1993: 151). Dr. Joseph Jones, a Confederate doctor, estimated that each of the Confederate soldiers fell ill about six times during the course of the war (Breeden 1975, cited in Duffy 1993: 152). Union soldiers, who were better fed and supplied, suffered an average of two bouts of illness per soldier. Undoubtedly, the figures for either Confederate or Union forces underestimate the scale of illness impacts.

If it had not been evident early in the Civil War, the Battle of Shiloh (April 6–7, 1862) certainly made clear the need for medical care both in the Union and Confederate homelands, and on the brutal front lines where the forces met. Not only were there 23,000 casualties, but there were 8,400 wounded Union soldiers and 8,000 wounded Confederate soldiers from that battle. The Union Army had suffered a surprise attack and there were no field hospitals; in fact, much of the surgery occurred adjacent to the battle (Humphreys 2013: 34). The necessity of transporting wounded soldiers away from the front lines became apparent at Shiloh, and even more apparent at Richmond later in the spring and summer of 1862.

Organizing Medical Relief: Hospitals

After a rather slow realization of the scale of medical needs during the war, the Union Army put Dr. William A. Hammond into the position of Surgeon General on April 25, 1862 (Adams 1996: 31–32). In some regards, Hammond was the perfect person for the job. He had served eleven years already as a military surgeon, and had then served as professor of medicine at the University of Maryland. Hammond's strength, many said, was his vision of reforming medical care for the Union Army. His installation of a number of medical directors ensured that Hammond could immediately begin instituting changes in the procedures for combat surgery and care.

Hammond hired about 300 surgeons in addition to those already serving and appointed a number of able medical instructors and specialists to assist with instituting reforms. He asked for ambulances and ambulance personnel. He advocated for increased rank and pay for army surgeons. One of his most important contributions was that he introduced the pavilion hospital design for army hospitals as well as the "ridge ventilation" system to provide fresh air. In order to maximize ventilation and minimize density of patient atmospheric sharing, the pavilion design created hospitals that stretched out horizontally and emphasized physical separation of wards.

The internal pavilion hospital structure was designed to minimize contact between patient rooms and the clinical and domestic areas. Windows and doors were to be placed so as to maximize air flow and sunlight. Height was limited to one or two stories. Pavilion hospitals had a central portion, often with administrative offices, with wings that extended beyond the central portion in various directions (Figure 6.1). The design allowed for both the segregation of patients according to their medical conditions and for the proper ventilation of the wards (Adams 1966; Duffy 1993: 156).

As discussed by Thompson and Goldin (1975) in their extensive review of hospital design, both physical and social, most hospitals prior to the mid-nineteenth century were not designed with sanitation in mind. The pavilion hospital changed that:

> The pavilion, however, when used for wards is a sanitary code embodied in a building. Pavilion in this sense means an open ward, but of limited extent; ventilated on both long sides by windows, on both

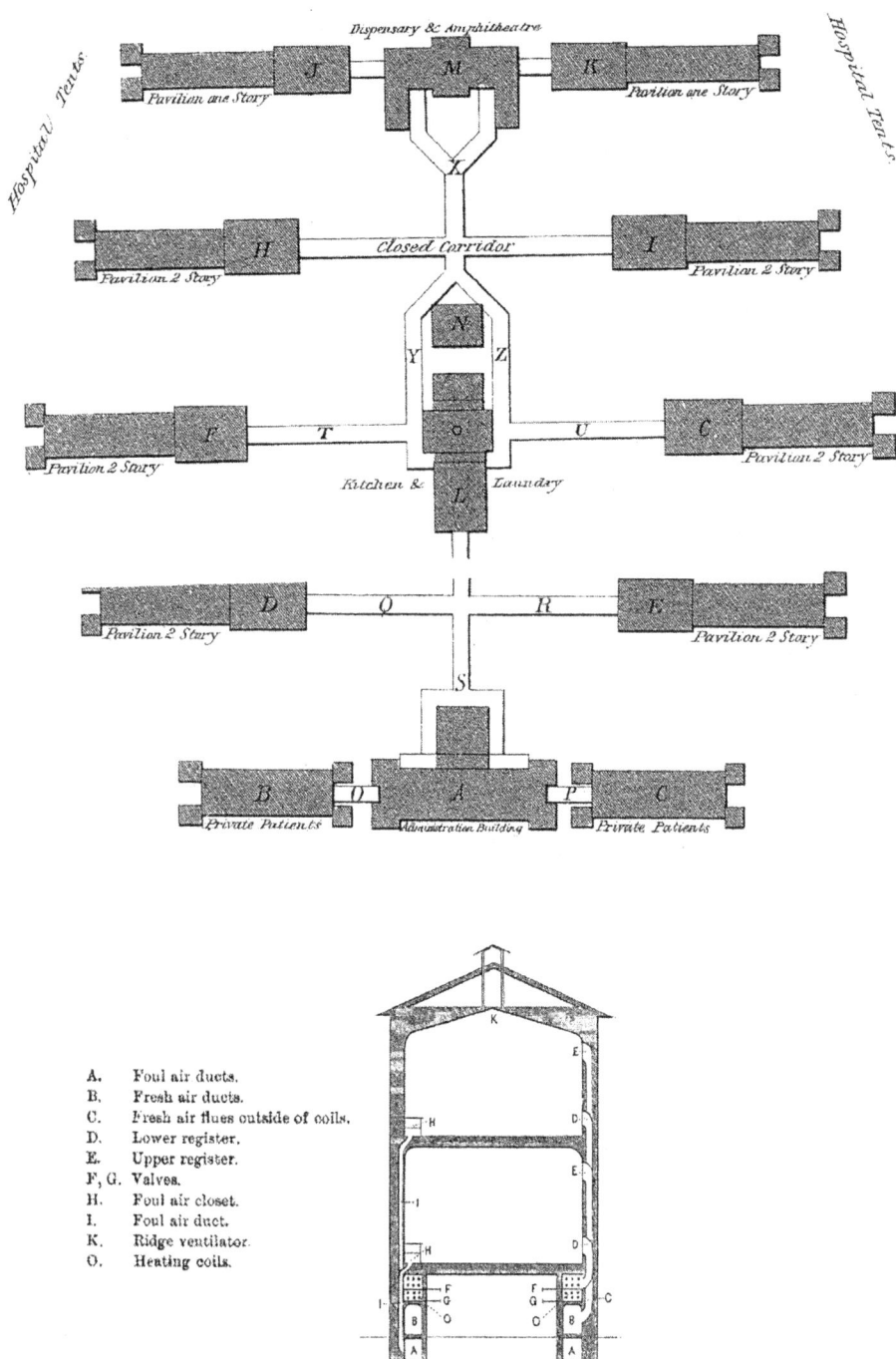

Figure 6.1. Typical pavilion hospital building plan. Billings' Plan Number 5 for Johns Hopkins Hospital (*top*) with two-story ridge ventilation (*bottom*). Adapted from Billings 1875a, pages 30 and 53.

short sides by doors; connected to a corridor that served similar pavilions, but self-contained with its own service rooms. This type of ward came into use in the middle of the nineteenth century, and the last examples are only vanishing now. For a hundred years the pavilion was the dominant ward form. (Thompson and Goldin 1975: 118)

Two types of hospitals were established during the Civil War: the field hospital and the general hospital. General hospitals, if newly constructed, were largely built in the pavilion plan and were located far behind the lines of battle. They provided care for the most seriously wounded, or those faced with long-term recovery. Soldiers had to be transported from the battlefront to general hospitals, which occurred largely by ship or train. Field hospitals were located near the battlefront and provided the initial medical treatment for the wounded or ill. It was there that those with recoverable ailments such as diarrhea could mend, or those requiring immediate treatment such as amputations could receive medical aid.

Satterlee Hospital (originally West Philadelphia Hospital) is a perfect example of Hammond's oversight of large general hospital construction in the pavilion style during the Civil War (Figure 6.2). Like many of the earlier hospitals, it was situated adjacent to the urban center on undeveloped land. It was built in a matter of five months, although the first patients were moved into six wards after only a month and a half.

When it was completed, Satterlee consisted of 28 wards, each which would accommodate 70 patients. There was a chapel, library, dining hall, smoking room, and a billiard table. The entire complex boasted several other buildings that included kitchens, a laundry, staff and guard quarters, a post office, and a storage building for 3,000 backpacks and personal possessions (Humphreys 2013). It was virtually a small city located on fifteen acres that could additionally accommodate hundreds of tents. The main hospital building was later enlarged and could provide 4,500 beds.

Hammond hired Isaac Hayes, a doctor trained in medicine at the University of Pennsylvania, to run the hospital. Hayes was better known as a traveler to the Arctic and a naturalist. With Hayes at the helm, West Philadelphia Hospital was up and running in forty days with an impressive set of facilities. Each ward had an iron stove and ventilation through roof vents, hot water, a water closet, and bathing facilities (Figure 6.3). There was an efficient kitchen and laundry. Twelve pharmacists oversaw the provisioning of pharmaceuticals, and there were 40 physicians and another 40 medical students as assistants.

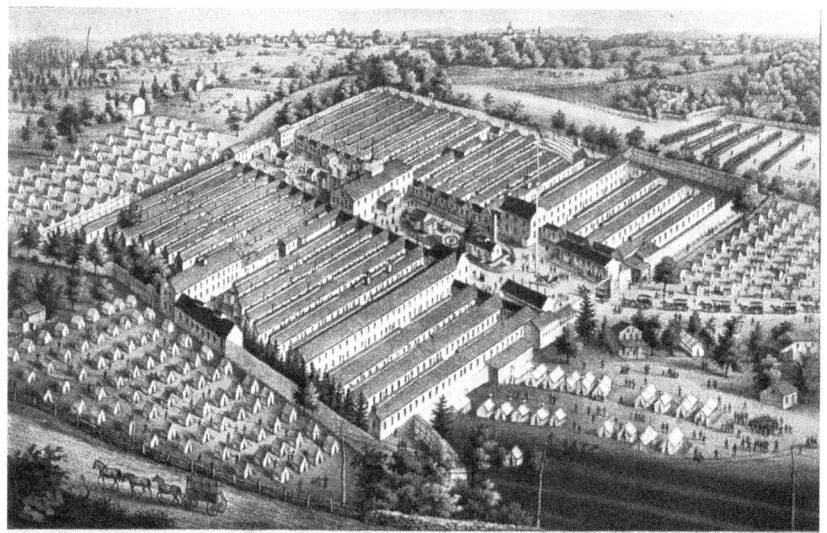

Figure 6.2. Satterlee Hospital. Lithograph by Charles Magnus. Lithograph, color, National Library of Medicine Unique ID: 101394053 (see catalog record), NLM Image ID: A024127.

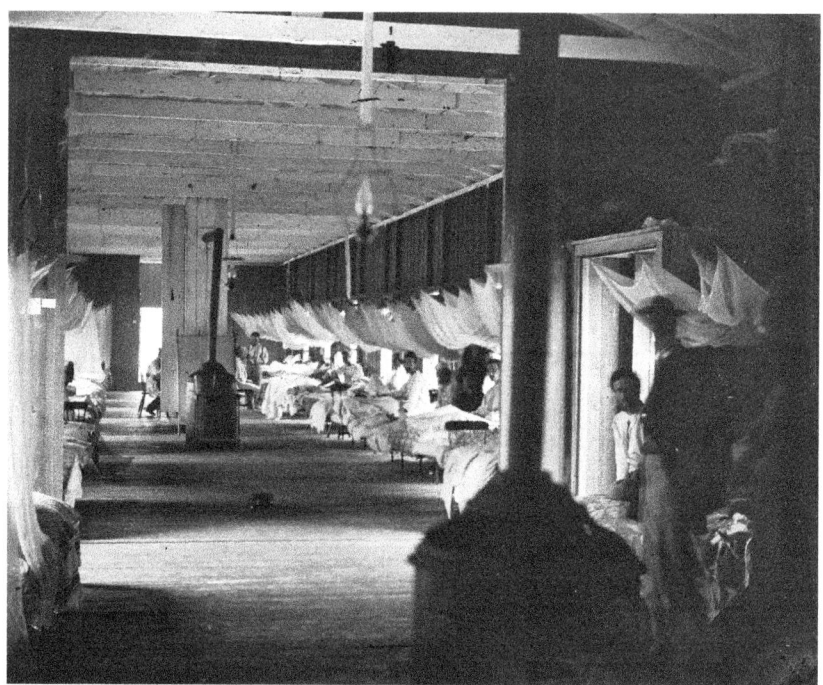

Figure 6.3. Patients at Harewood Hospital in Washington, DC, 1864. Civil war photographs, 1861–1865, Courtesy of Library of Congress, Prints and Photographs Division. Reproduction Number: LC-DIG-cwpb-00485 (digital file from original neg.).

The largest hospital to be constructed using the pavilion plan was the Confederate Chimborazo Hospital in Richmond; it was, in fact, the largest hospital in the world at the time of the Civil War (Cunningham 1958): "At one point it consisted of some one hundred small buildings, long narrow rectangles of rough wood eighty feet long by twenty-eight feet wide with seven-foot-high walls. Each long wall had ten windows, and there were doors at both ends and in the middle. These were ideal structures for ventilation (although difficult to heat in winter), and the air space for patients was jealously guarded" (Humphreys 2013: 85).

The regular placement of people into hospitals made the Civil War unique. Prior to the war, only the indigent and poor, or those in the maritime trades, were sent to hospitals; those in the upper and middle classes were provided care at home. The war changed that, and whatever station a person held prior to the war did not matter with regard to hospitalization; if you were wounded or sick, you went to a hospital.

Organizing Medical Relief: Front Lines

Surgeon General Hammond recognized the need for battlefield transport of the wounded, but he received little support from Congress or Secretary of War Edwin M. Stanton. Ambulance transport was novel at the time of the Civil War, and although some ambulances were supplied, they and their staff were inadequate. At the Battle of Bull Run in July 1861, for instance, ambulances were driven by civilians who abandoned the wounded as they retreated (Adams 1996: 26; Duffy 1993: 157).

Hammond, however, persisted in his cause. Again, his vision of capable medical directors was fulfilled by Jonathan Letterman as Medical Director of the Army of the Potomac in July of 1862. Letterman quickly began to implement reforms in how the wounded were provided care. One of those reforms was the establishment of an ambulance unit to be assigned to each regiment, with people and wagons assigned to quickly move the wounded away from the battlefront. His reorganization of the ambulance service and his reorganization of the field hospital system were well recognized (Adams 1996; Freeman 2001).

Letterman also personally inspected the Union camps and found that dietary-deficiency diseases, especially scurvy (vitamin C deficiency), were common. He ordered that the usual diet provided to the troops of pork or beef, bread or crackers, beans, rice, and coffee be supplemented with fresh vegetables, potatoes, and onions. Letterman also recognized that hospitals needed even more nutritious foods if soldiers were to recover from their wounds. Nonetheless, transport problems to some areas of the war, combined with officers diverting the fresh foods for their own use, often meant that shortages of fresh produce still occurred and dietary deficiencies were maintained.

In addition to malnutrition, the camps were the location of major sanitary problems and diseases both of sanitation and aggregation. Measles, smallpox, and other crowd diseases were common in Union forces, but Confederates were even more susceptible. Northern soldiers were often from urban areas and were thus more frequently exposed as children to many, if not all, crowd diseases. The vast majority of Southerners, on the other hand, were from rural areas with less childhood crowd-disease experience.

Gastrointestinal diseases of sanitation such as diarrhea, dysentery, and typhoid were frequent in the camps of both forces. The Union Army, for instance, recorded 215,214 cases of diarrhea and dysentery between 1861 and 1862 (Duffy 1993: 159). Malaria was endemic in the South and commonly affected the troops, although distinguishing it from other fevers was sometimes challenging and thus the phrase "typho-malaria" was commonly used. Respiratory disorders plagued both forces with a mortality rate for pneumonia of about 20 percent (Duffy 1993: 160).

The Confederate Medical Department was headed by Surgeon General Samuel Preston Moore, equally as visionary as Hammond. He also appointed able colleagues; one of them, Samuel Stout, instituted many of the same reforms for transport and field hospitals as Letterman (Duffy 1993: 159). The South initially had a more efficient railroad transport system for the wounded, but as the war went on it became overused, and there were fewer alternative vehicles or animals for transport in the South.

There were advantages and disadvantages to the fact that the Confederate Army was fighting in their homeland. While geographic familiarity was an advantage, the Confederate homeland soon became a war-torn landscape. Shortages of food for Confederate soldiers, however, were met by civilian support, unlike that for the Northern army, which had to transport their food into the front lines.

One could not do justice to a discussion of medical care during the Civil War without recognizing the immense role of female medical practitioners (Schultz 2004). Many people have heard of Clara Barton, who organized battlefield relief stations, and many recognize the immense number of women who served as nurses. Jane Schultz, a historian, found references to more than 22,000 female hospital workers during the war in the pension records of the National Archives and other places (Schultz 2004: 20–21). Neither the Union nor Confederate armies, however, took much advantage of women in the role of physicians. There were over 200 women at the time of the Civil War who were formally trained and had obtained an MD degree (Humphreys 2013: 54).

Most women who tried to attain roles as physicians were turned down, but at least three were able to serve in that capacity. The most famous was Mary Edwards Walker, who served as a contract physician for the Fifty-Second Ohio Regiment in 1864. Her stint in that capacity was short as she was captured by the Confederate Army only two months after she began her post. Following her release, she worked another year or so in other capacities in the military, but her relationships with male physicians were apparently highly contentious. Nonetheless, in November 1865 she received the Congressional Medal of Honor for her wartime activities from President Andrew Johnson.

Organizing Medical Relief: Surgery and Amputation

The scale of traumatic injury during the Civil War was unprecedented. About 94 percent of all wounds suffered during the Civil War were caused by bullets, and they were not a type of trauma that most surgeons had experienced prior to the war. The expansive bullet (minie ball) was a conical ball with a hollow base which tended to flatten on contact while shattering the bone and dragging clothing and other debris into the wound. This would frequently result in infection (Freeman 2001). The Battle of Gettysburg, for instance, left more than 14,500 Union soldiers and 7,300 in the Confederate Army wounded (Humphreys 2013:39).

Amputation was the major way of treating bullet wounds as it resulted in a higher rate of survival than delayed surgery. More amputations occurred in the Civil War than any other conflict involving America, approximately 60,000 (Figg and Farrell-Beck 1993: 454). Roughly 75 percent of all operations were amputations (Brooks 1966: 97; Cunningham 1958: 225). However, the practice of amputation was not without debate. It was seen by some as going against a trend in "conservative medicine" (for example, splinting and excision), which often resulted in complications such as infection or ankylosis (stiffening, sometimes fusion) of the joints.

Antiseptic surgery, which was stressed as important by Surgeon General Hammond, was still not always practiced, especially early in the war. When infection did occur, a number of physicians interpreted the formation of pus as part of the normal healing process. Most of the time they let the infection go until it became severely inflamed or the patient developed gangrene (Duffy 1993: 162).

There was also no uniform acceptance of anesthesia—it was distrusted by those advocating less "heroic" medical intervention. Yet, it was clearly often employed by some doctors, as indicated by the numerous syringes found in the excavations at Dr. Clifford Morrogh's home and office in New Brunswick, New Jersey (Veit 1996; see Chapter 5). While those syringes may have been used for some other purpose, the fact that Dr. Morrogh was a pioneer in the use of anesthesia, combined with the well-documented use of morphine sulfate injection for anesthesia, supports their use for such a purpose.

Several lancets were also found at the Morrogh property, which were likely used to aid syringe injection. The use of lancets was in decline, as was bleeding, by the mid-nineteenth century, but lancets were also widely used for opening an injection site. Until 1853 when Alexander Wood invented sharp, hollow hypodermic needles, it was common to use a lancet to open up a site for injection with a syringe (Veit 1996). Morphine injections became an important part of Civil War battlefield surgery to relieve pain (Flannery 2017: 116). It was not delivered solely by injection though: "A great advantage which they [the salts of morphine] possess is the convenience of their external application to blistered surfaces, and the certainty of their effects when thus applied" (Formento 1863: 49).

Anesthesia, while available in the form of chloroform and ether, was fairly unfamiliar to many doctors, who had few occasions to use it given the relative absence of surgical experience. Chloroform, first introduced only in 1847, was the preferred method of anesthesia as it was nonflammable, and it was simply dripped onto a cloth and placed over the patient's face (Devine 2014; Figure 6.4). Deaths from anesthesia ranged between 3 per 1,000 for ether, to 5.4 per 1,000 for chloroform (Duffy 1993: 162).

Given the above concerns, whether to amputate and when were of some discussion. If amputation was the chosen path for a wound, there was general agreement in both the Union and Confederate armies that it be done relatively soon after the wound occurred. Federal classifications of surgical timing were standardized: primary (within 48 hours), intermediate (days 3 to 30), and secondary (after the 30th day when inflammation had subsided) (Otis and Huntington 1883: 878). Intermediate amputations had the highest mortality rate, at 35 percent. Primary amputations had the lowest mortality rate, at 24 percent, with secondary amputations slightly higher, at 29 percent (Otis and Huntington 1883: 879).

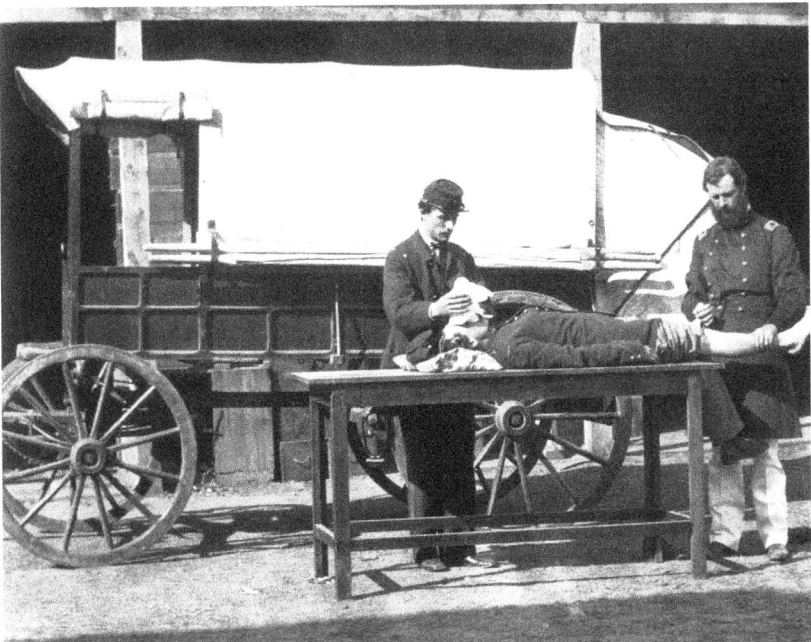

Figure 6.4. Administration of anesthesia. Posed photograph showing how anesthesia was dripped onto a sponge or cone that fit over the nose and mouth of the patient. Note the rudimentary table on which surgery is to be performed and the medical ambulance. Courtesy National Museum of Health and Medicine. "Army Medical Wagon" (CP 1563). OHA 75 Contributed Photographs Collection. Otis Historical Archives, National Museum of Health and Medicine.

It became apparent early in the Civil War that hygiene and disinfection were of paramount importance. Medical personnel recognized the importance of cleansing wounds quickly, and it was one important function of field hospitals. Elisha Harris, a Union physician, highlighted the importance of disinfectants to neutralize "poisons" that cause disease in a pamphlet called *Control and Prevention of Infectious Diseases* (Humphreys 2013: 80). Topical disinfectants were almost universally used on wounds after 1862 and included bromine, iodine, and nitric acid. Antiseptic treatment of wounds with gangrene also occurred using iodine, bromine, and chlorine, carbolic and nitric acid, and turpentine, but often they were administered too many days into the time of the infection.

Certainly the widespread use of disinfectants prevented more than a few cases of gangrene. Unfortunately, many commonly used medicines were of mixed effectiveness and largely functioned as purgatives and emetics.

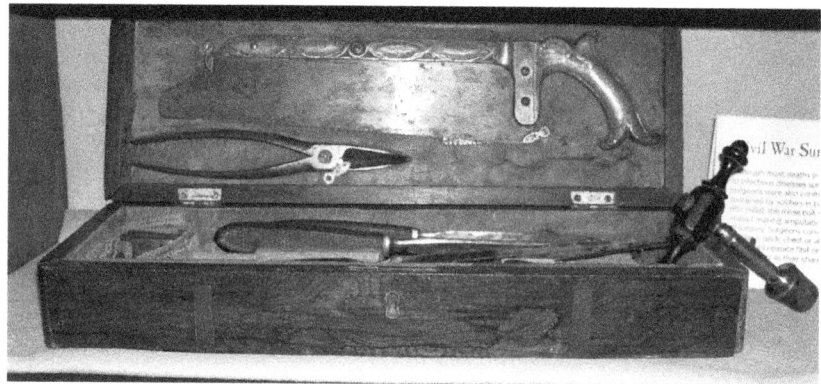

Figure 6.5. Surgical kit typical of a field physician. Photographed by the author at the Country Doctor Museum, Bailey, NC.

Those commonly prescribed were calomel (mercurous chloride), tartar emetic (antimony), opiates, various mercury compounds, alcohol, and quinine. The use of calomel, although very common, was also heavily debated; it acted as a laxative and caused the patient to salivate. It was one of the main ingredients cited in Surgeon General Hammond's court-martial (see below), as he forbade its use.

The success of amputation was hampered by a number of factors. One was simply the scale of battle wounds; at Gettysburg, surgeons spent an entire week amputating limbs (Brooks 1966: 97). A second was the limited surgical kit of the physician in the field, which contained a selection of probes, tourniquets, scalpels, and saws for conducting amputations and other surgeries, but little else (Figure 6.5). There was initially a complete absence of the kinds of medical technology that were well established in France; stethoscopes, thermometers, syringes, ophthalmoscopes, and laryngoscopes were well entrenched in hospitals by the end of the Civil War, but not at the beginning.

Thousands of wounded soldiers lived following amputations of some of their limbs or other body parts (Bengston and Kuz 1996). Otis and Huntington's chapter in the surgery volume of *Medical and Surgical History of the War of the Rebellion* (1883: 869) states that 21,753 patients survived the 29,980 amputations that were performed (73 percent). Consequently, prosthetic limbs were widely distributed and a familiar sight for a generation following the war.

Dr. George Otis supervised the photographic documentation of many of the individuals who had suffered amputations (Figure 6.6). In the earliest

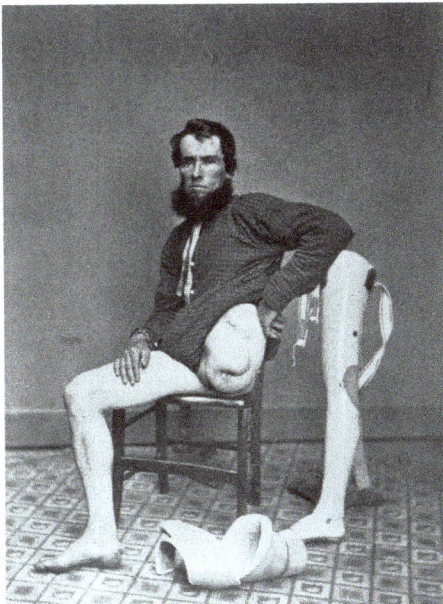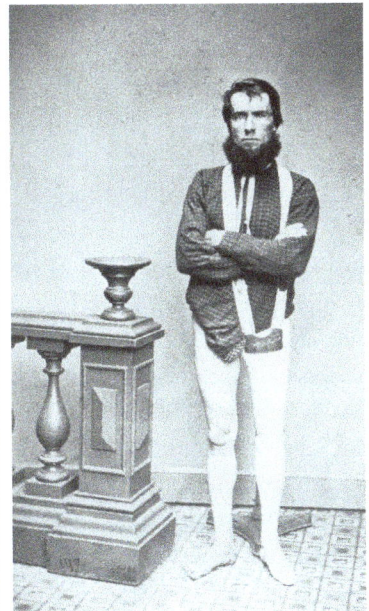

Figure 6.6. Successful amputation of the left hip joint and prosthesis for Private James E. Kelley, 56th Pennsylvania Regiment, age 28 when wounded. Case of successful primary amputation at the hip-joint (SP 196). OHA 82 Surgical Photographs Collection. Otis Historical Archives, National Museum of Health and Medicine (*left*). Case of successful primary amputation at the hip-joint, wearing prosthesis (SP 197). OHA 82 Surgical Photographs Collection. Otis Historical Archives, National Museum of Health and Medicine (*right*).

years of documentation, the photographs were taken by William Bell at his nearby studio, and thus they look more like studio photographs than ones taken for medical purposes (Rhode 1996, vi).

Between 1861 and 1873, 133 patents were issued for prosthetic limbs, an increase of 290 percent from the fifteen years prior to the war (Figg and Farrell-Beck 1993: 460). Veterans who had survived amputations were eligible for government pensions and subsidies for artificial limbs, but only if they fought for the Union Army. In 1862, the year the Act of 16 July was passed, an amputee could receive $50 to purchase a prosthetic arm or foot and $75 for a leg (Figg and Farrell-Beck 1993: 463).

Much credit for the success of medical treatment of Union soldiers during the Civil War is undoubtedly due to Surgeon General Hammond. He was an energetic and visionary reformer, but unfortunately he irritated many people, especially his superior, Secretary of War Stanton. His

"Circular 6," issued in the spring of 1863, demanded the removal of two dangerous but popular drugs, Calomel and Tartar emetic, from the army medical supply table. The responses were mixed. The botanics and sectarians heralded his order as medical progress. For his allopathic colleagues, however, his order went too far and he was arrested to face court-martial, largely on trumped-up charges.

Hammond was indeed found guilty and ushered out of the medical corps, but only after most of his reforms were in place. He was replaced by Joseph K. Barnes who closed out the war. When Joseph K. Barnes took over the Surgeon General's office in 1864 following Hammond's dismissal, he reorganized the office staff. Among the people he added were George A. Otis and John Shaw Billings. Billings was put in charge of the library of the Surgeon General's Office and would do much later to influence hospital reform (Freeman 2001: 160).

There was one other consequence of the tremendous mortality suffered in the Civil War. Many families of dead soldiers wanted the bodies of their loved ones back for burial, perhaps to see their beloved family members one more time, and they turned to embalmers to aid in the preservation of the body. Embalming was not a standard part of mortuary treatment prior to the war, and was used almost exclusively in America by medical schools to preserve corpses for dissection. It was done by injection of chemical preservative (Figures 6.7–6.8) into an artery (usually the femoral). It was not cheap for Civil War families—$50 for an officer ($1,017 in today's currency) and $25 for an enlisted soldier ($509 in today's currency) (Devine 2014: 177). Thus, it was reserved primarily for families with money while those less privileged were buried hastily at the battlefront.

* * *

The health and well-being consequences of the Civil War went beyond wounds, illnesses, amputations, and death. The hostilities between the North and South also included the incarceration of prisoners of war. At the end of the war in 1865, 32 Union Army and 33 Confederate Army penal compounds had been constructed and they held approximately 420,000 prisoners over the four-year war (Bush 2000: 64; Hesseltine 1930: 2). Archaeological investigations at several Civil War penal institutions have taken place over the past 45 years (Bush 2000; Casella 2007; Prentice and Prentice 2000; Thoms 2004).

Andersonville prison in western Georgia was established on 16.5 acres surrounded by swamp and was enclosed in a stockade. Three stages of

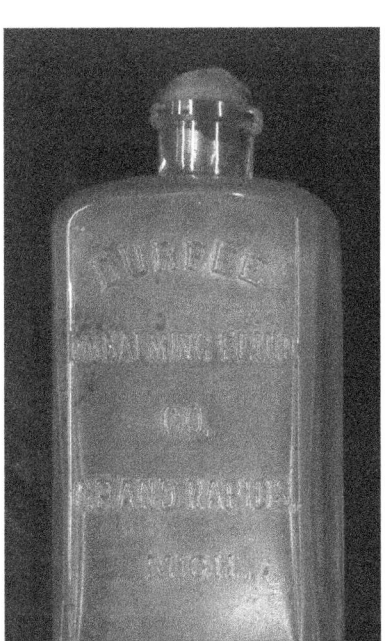 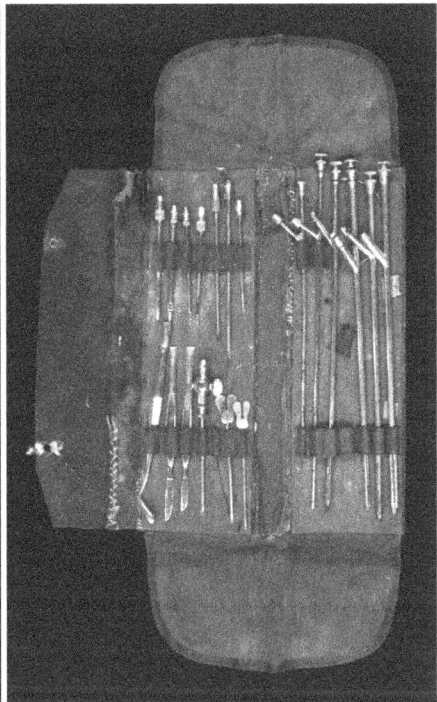

Left: Figure 6.7. Embalming fluid bottle. From the collection of embalmer David E. Wolfe, courtesy of Mr. Wolfe; photographed by Cheney J. Schopieray, William L. Clements Library, University of Michigan, Ann Arbor.

Right: Figure 6.8. Embalming kit. From the collection of embalmer David E. Wolfe, courtesy of Mr. Wolfe; photographed by Cheney J. Schopieray, William L. Clements Library, University of Michigan, Ann Arbor. The original owner of the embalming kit was Lowell M. Clapp, Kalkaska, MI, undertaker from 1907 to 1935.

archaeological investigation had been conducted by 1990, and they revealed the stockade, building foundations, and an escape tunnel (Bearss 1970; Larson and Crook 1975; Prentice and Prentice 2000). Although originally designed to accommodate 10,000 prisoners, the incarcerated population of Union soldiers rapidly grew to 23,000. Crowding was an issue. Historical accounts report that there were insufficient clean water, food, medicine, and blankets (Bearss 1970: 147).

In order to address the larger population, the walls were extended to include 25 acres, the labor provided by the undernourished Union soldiers. Within months, the number of prisoners reached 33,000 men and the prison was once again marked by crowding, poor living conditions, and insufficient food and water. By the end of the war, Andersonville had seen the deaths of 12,290 prisoners as recorded by the hospital clerk.

The prisoners were not without agency, however. Excavations in the southeast corner of the Andersonville stockade revealed the remains of an escape tunnel. Running along the stockade wall, apparently the tunnel had to be aborted when several stockade posts collapsed into it before the tunnel could be completed (Prentice and Prentice 2000: 185).

The military prison at Johnson's Island presents a somewhat different picture than Andersonville. Established in 1862 as a Union prison for Confederate officers, accommodations and material culture indicate the more tolerable living conditions afforded the southern elite (Casella 2007). It was located on western Lake Erie in Ohio and, like Andersonville, had a stockade wall. Most of the archaeological research was focused on latrine features, from which a number of material culture items were found.

Letters from the prisoners, as well as material culture, document the declining Union support of POW camps after 1863 and the impacts that decline had on the Johnson's Island prisoners. Prior to 1863, there appears to have been sufficient food. After 1863, letters and food remains document increasingly supplemental food sources such as rabbit, rodent, bird, dog, and fish (Casella 2007: 124). Material culture also indicates the reduction in medical support after 1863 (Bush 2000). Analysis of the glass recovered from the hospital latrines clearly documents a reduction in pharmaceutical bottles (those provisioned by the army hospital) and an increase in patent medicine bottles (those purchased by the soldiers). Regardless of the type of medicine container, both types of containers decline in frequency in 1864 (Bush 2000).

* * *

Nestled in a corner of the northern part of the District of Columbia once stood a museum called the Armed Forces Medical Museum, and an associated research and curatorial facility called the Armed Forces Institute of Pathology (AFIP). The AFIP housed the physical remains, testimonials, and photographs of thousands of Civil War soldiers. It had its humble beginnings in Surgeon General William Hammond's office; it was Hammond who in another visionary moment issued orders to establish the Army Medical Museum (Stone 2011: 3).

It was the material collected during the Civil War that formed the primary data for the *Medical and Surgical History of the War of the Rebellion* (MSHW). George A. Otis, one of the section authors of the MSHW, was the second curator of the museum from 1864 until 1881. His coauthor on the surgical section of the MSHW, David Low Huntington, was the third curator from 1881 to 1883.

John Shaw Billings, another instrumental figure in armed forces medicine, was the fourth curator from 1883 until 1893. Billings was an energetic curator, and during his decade in that position he moved the emphasis of the museum beyond anatomical specimens in America to a more global focus, and incorporated the material culture of medicine (Stone 2011: 30). It was Billings who persisted in demanding more space in which the medical staff could expand both their collections and their endeavors.

Billings was ultimately successful, and the museum moved to the larger building in 1887 and stayed there for 80 years. He was succeeded by no less a formidable fifth curator than Major Walter Reed in 1893. In his ten-year career at the museum, Reed not only championed its causes, but expanded them in the direction of experimenting with X-rays after their discovery in 1896. He headed an army board to investigate how typhoid fever spreads in camps, and in another assignment headed the investigative team in Cuba that discovered how yellow fever is transmitted.

I mention the names of the curators because many of them were dedicated to not only preserving the medical legacy of the Civil War, but had major impacts on the development of the hospital system and other important issues of hygiene beyond the military, as Woodward states below. They made sure that what they had been taught by the Civil War did not go forgotten. I had the honor to visit the AFIP collections to conduct research on two occasions early in my career, and I can honestly say those visits left a lasting impression on me and contributed immensely to both my teaching and research. Unfortunately, the AFIP closed its doors in 2011 and the collections and functions have been dispersed to other facilities (Stone 2011).

> There can be no doubt the [Civil War] has given great impetus to medical study in America, and this is not merely the directive of operative surgery and public hygiene, on which its effect has been perhaps the most obvious, but in many collateral branches also on some of which a favorable influence from this source could scarcely have been anticipated. (Woodward 1871: 233)

* * *

Many medical historians credit the advances made in public health after 1860 to the emphasis of Civil War doctors on antiseptic surgery and laboratory work. The war stimulated changes in how medical training occurred by creating the need for laboratory work in addition to lectures, and in the training of gross anatomy; by 1881 sixteen states had passed laws that permitted the use of unclaimed bodies to teach anatomy (Devine 2014: 7). By 1913, every state with a medical school had passed laws permitting the use of indigent cadavers for teaching anatomy except Alabama, Louisiana, Tennessee, and North Carolina (Sappol 2002: 5).

7

Ventilation, Germs, and Hygiene

The Post–Civil War Reform

> But certain it is new comers seldom pass July and August without a burning fever, which through intemperate drinking of water often draws after it the fluxe or dropsy, and where many are sick together, is infectious: This requires a skilful Physician, convenient diet and lodging with diligent attendance, few dying of the first brunt of sickness, but upon relapses for want of strengthening diet and good drink to repair the loss of that blood, which is taken from them. . . .
>
> (Wyatt, Letter of Sir Francis 1926: 117)

Early in the colonial period, the simplicity of hygiene, or so it seemed, was ensured by digging pits, some for depositing bodily wastes and some for supplying water. Such was the case in Jamestown, Virginia, as Wyatt reports. Settled in 1607 on the James River, a well was dug in late 1608 or early 1609 which was lined with a barrel. It descended to a depth of 14 feet, and appears to have been used only a couple of years until 1611. John Smith recorded that "we digged a faire Well of fresh water in the Fort of excellent, sweet water which till then was wanting" (Smith 1629: 101).

By May of 1610, the secretary of the colony, William Strachey, recorded that "James Town . . . hath no fresh water springs serving town but what we drew from a well six or seven fathom deep, fed by the brackish river oozing into it; from whence I verily believe the chief causes have proceeded of many diseases and sicknesses which have happened to our people, who indeed are strangely afflicted with fluxes and agues, and every particular infirmity too" (Strachey 1610: 82). The well had become contaminated with human wastes that were unable to percolate beneath the saltwater.

With the growth of population in the colonial period, especially for those living in urban centers, hygiene became even more of a problem (Rothschild and Wall 2014). Concerns over hygiene encompassed several areas of health and well-being. Animal wastes were always an issue, human and otherwise, and much of the time water served as a vehicle for cleaning up the wastes. Then it was no longer clean. Keeping dirty water from mingling with clean water was a constant struggle, again especially in cities.

It was not just water sanitation that was an issue, but anything that became stressed with aggregation, and the colonization of America was all about aggregation. Population density, whether in rural or urban environments, was increasing decade by decade. It didn't happen immediately, and it didn't happen universally for every geographic locality, but it did increasingly become a problem during the colonial process. Beyond water, there was the quality of air, contagion in proximity of infectious disease, and the organic and inorganic discards of a rapidly increasing population.

Most importantly, why people got sick and suffered from ill health, was scarcely understood until the late nineteenth century. Even when the causes were apparent, some segments of society had much more ability to avoid problematic situations than others. And so, for a couple of hundred years, people struggled with containing wastes, providing clean water, and maintaining clean air. It wasn't easy.

Designing Defecation Disposal

Whether it was called a toilet, cesspit, water closet, chamber pot, john, latrine, loo, necessary, porcelain god, lavatory, latrine, cloakroom, smallest room, closet, commode, chamber of commerce, house of office, privy, crapper, or outhouse, that special facility or unit to utilize for one's bodily functions has a very long and colorful history reaching well back beyond the Roman Empire. Before privies, and indeed alongside their use, there were chamber pots dumped of their contents outside, and barrels in the ground.

While there is no central plan for privy construction, there are some common features. They generally have three walls and a fourth has a door. There is an elevated platform with a hole for depositing one's offerings. Sometimes there is a seat around that hole, and sometimes a cover for the hole and seat. There can be a single hole or multiple, and the multiple holes can be of different sizes to accommodate the younger and smaller contributors.

Beyond those criteria stands much variation, mostly in how the contents are treated following deposition. One method is to have an opening at the bottom and the contents simply become accessible, often with the thought that some scavenging animal will take care of them; hogs are a common accomplice. In urban localities like New York, the deposits simply run out through foundation openings. In more rural localities, the outhouse can be placed strategically so that automatic reconfiguration of the deposits takes place. For example, one could locate the structure so that it projected partially over a ravine, with the contents simply dropping from the structure into the ravine. A colleague provided me with this example, and assures me that the user is frequently greeted in the process of making a deposit by the sounds of enthusiastic swine below, waiting for things to drop.

A second is to have a pit, generally 3 to 6 feet deep, which is periodically covered with dirt and perhaps lime. Once the pit is full, the outhouse is simply moved over a new pit. More elaborate designs include draining the contents off, usually in combination with a water "flush," to some other location, perhaps a creek, river, or cesspool. Whatever method is used to contain and eventually distribute the contents, privies have offensive odors and attract numerous insects, particularly flies. In the heat of summer, historical accounts report people feeling nauseous while close to privies.

Consider New York as an example of hygiene challenges. Originally settled in 1625 by the Dutch and named New Amsterdam, by 1650 there were already numerous sanitation problems. Like many emerging urban centers, wells and privies in early New Amsterdam were often private. The first nine public wells in New York were built in 1677 after the English took charge of the city in 1664, and all were brackish (Duffy 1968: 30). The best sources of fresh water were springs and rivers, but the water from those sources had to be transported into the city. Some of the same saltwater contamination issues that were suffered by Jamestown were also present for New York. The constant tension between sources of fresh water, places to deposit human wastes, and places to dump refuse, both organic and inorganic, escalated through time.

Privies were not the only problem, but they certainly were major contributors. Many people left their privy outlet level with the ground and counted on hogs to take care of the materials deposited. Drainage of sewage into a centralized system was not really a concept in the seventeenth century; canals and drainage lines were mostly designed for groundwater drainage. There was neither any concept of separate kinds of drainage, nor the recognition that proper drainage required planning and maintenance. In 1657, for instance, a canal was deepened and widened to allow dockage and drainage. Called the *Heeregraft*, it soon became a popular place to dispose of dead animals, trash, and general refuse. By 1675, it had become so tainted with dead animals and refuse, it had to be backfilled.

From the time of the Heeregraft until the sanitary campaigns following 1860, animals were nearly as common as humans in New York; dogs, goats, pigs, even cows, wandered through the streets. Horses were the predominant mode of transport. Dead animals regularly adorned the street and remained commonplace for two centuries. "In May of 1853, for example, the City Inspector reported that 439 large dead animals had been removed from the streets along with the bodies of 71 dogs, 93 cats, 17 sheep, 4 goats, and 19 hogs" (Duffy 1968: 57).

The traffic of animals in New York simply added to the problems of public hygiene in the streets. Yet over the years, humans and animals, especially hogs, came to a set of understandings about each of their roles vis-à-vis privies. It was not a set of roles embraced by everyone, and privies were a nuisance in New York for a couple of centuries. They were supposed to be cleaned, but service was irregular. A series of "privy laws" were enacted throughout New York during the 1600s and 1700s to combat the rising volume and smell. In 1658, New York City officials ordered that all privies with their outlets even with the ground had to be removed:

> WHEREAS many, even the greatest part of the burghers and inhabitants of this City build their privies even with the ground with an opening towards the street, so that hogs may consume the filth and wallow in it, which not only creates a great stench and therefore great inconvenience to the passers-by, but also makes the streets foul and unfit for use,-therefore. . . . the Burgonmasters and Schepens, herewith order and command, that all and everybody. . . . shall break down and remove such privies coming out upon the street. (*Records of New Amsterdam*, I, 31, quoted in Duffy 1968: 18)

City officials and health officers would struggle with enforcing that edict for over a century and numerous privy laws would be put forth. Privies would continue to be the primary toilet facility for at least a century, and for archaeologists at least, that was a good thing.

Despite their many problems, privies are embraced by archaeologists. Quite simply, privies are a window into the past. They harbor secrets, both by purposeful inclusion and by accident. Archaeologists are especially fond of excavating privies because of their function as receptacles for all sorts of material culture. Many privies were well maintained and periodically capped with lime or some other sealing material which contained the smells of one level and served as a floor for the deposition and olfactory vapors of the next (Carnes-McNaugton and Harper 2000; Heck and Balicki

1998). Those periods of maintenance often allow for nicely stratified deposits of archaeological materials. Frequently, the terminal event was a filling of the remaining pit feature, often with lots of material culture. Later intrusion and removal of materials seldom occurs until archaeologists come along.

Katherine Naylor's house offers a perfect example of privy accumulation of rich deposits (Heck and Balicki 1998). Katherine occupied the house between roughly 1650 and 1700 with two different husbands and two children. Excavations between 1990 and 1992 of Katherine's property (now the Cross Street Back Lot site in Boston) revealed a brick-lined vault designated Feature 4 and determined to be a privy. The deposits indicate the privy was used primarily during the last quarter of the seventeenth century. Fairly constant waterlogged conditions provided an anaerobic environment that allowed the preservation of flora and fauna, shell, textile, wood, and leather materials.

Several periods of privy use were each followed by episodes of cleaning, construction, maintenance, and fill deposition. Among the material items recovered from the deposits were tin-glazed earthenwares, clay pipes, spoons and other tableware, a complete redware chamber pot, a brass bucket, leather shoe parts, textiles, sewing tools, a wooden lawn bowling ball, musket balls, textiles, and straight pins, to name just a few. In addition to material culture, there were faunal remains recovered, intestinal parasite eggs, and approximately 166,000 seeds (Heck and Balicki 1998).

Privies and intestinal parasites go together for obvious reasons, and the analysis of the parasites can tell us some interesting things. One of the things they can reveal is the intestinal health of the occupants that use a privy. Do the depositors recognize their parasite problems and attempt to medically or mechanically intervene? Do they cook their food well enough to kill the parasites, for instance, in the case of tapeworms? Do they have habits that expose them to intestinal parasites, such as not cleaning surfaces that are in contact with food, to prevent acquiring a case of roundworm eggs? Do improvements in water and sewage sanitation have an effect on parasite loads?

Intestinal parasites are acquired through a variety of mechanisms, ranging from ingestion of the eggs (for example, roundworm, *Ascaris lumbricoides*), to ingestion of the larvae (for example, beef tapeworm, *Taenia saginata*), to penetration of the feet (for example, hookworm, *Necator americanus*). The eggs are generally what archaeologists recover, and the species present in the deposits give us lots of information about human health and economy. Variation in species could be linked to dietary preference, cooking methods, and household economy. The presence of intestinal parasites also can aid in interpreting other compounds found in the privy deposits that may have been used for treatment. Briefly, the analytical protocols for parasite analysis are centered on collecting soil samples, cleaning off the samples to isolate the eggs, identifying those eggs as to genus and/or species, and counting them. A more inclusive discussion of methods can be found in Fisher et al. (2007: 175–176).

Among the most interesting things recovered from Katherine Naylor's house or office are intestinal parasite eggs of whipworms and roundworms that were found in several levels and probably indicate chronic intestinal infestations. The presence of floral and pollen remains suggests the use of medicinal plants for worm medicines, as well as for headaches, fever, constipation, and hemorrhoids.

In 1984, another set of privies and cisterns associated with four adjoining house lots in Greenwich Village were excavated by archaeologists. Privies and cisterns from the Sullivan site, as it was called, revealed many things about health and well-being between 1840 and 1900 (Howson 1993). The artifacts found at Sullivan Street give a number of insights into the health, class, and finance of the people who lived on the four home lots.

For instance, only 27 patent medicine bottles, largely of well-known brand names, were found in all the cisterns and privies. The small number of patent medicine bottles suggests that the families were financially sound enough to afford a physician's care. That suggestion is supported by the thirteen medicine bottles that would have been dispensed by a doctor, and the fact that one of the families was that of Dr. Robson (Howson 1993: 151). Other objects relating to health included nine syringes, both hypodermic and vaginal, soap dishes, toothbrushes with bone handles, a toothbrush holder and container for tooth powder, and a plate of false teeth.

In 1993, archaeologists excavated a privy associated with a nineteenth-century tenement in New York's Five Points District. Five Points was the location of some of the worst tenement housing conditions, and at 12 Orange Street (later renamed Baxter Street), the location of the privy, was a brothel (see Chapter 3). The earliest date that could be assigned to the privy deposits (*terminus post quem*) is 1840 and is based on ceramic and glass artifacts found in the privy's primary soil layers. It appears that the deposit dates to a fairly tight time span of three to four years, as the owner of the property, John Donahue, was convicted on October 30, 1843, of keeping a disorderly house of ill-repute (Yamin 2005: 7). Parasite analysis was part of the research design for the project.

Karl Reinhard (2000), a specialist in archaeologically recovered intestinal parasites, reported a few interesting findings on his analysis of 25 samples from Five Points. For one, there were no pork or beef tapeworm eggs found, indicating that the residents did not suffer trichinosis from undercooked meat. When there were roundworm eggs found, the number was fewer than expected given analyses from other urban areas, which suggests that the residents reduced the parasite load through some type of treatment. Finally, as sanitation improved through time, it does not seem those improvements affected intestinal parasite loads. Samples at the top of the privy have about the same number of parasites as those at the bottom.

In another analysis, from Albany, Reinhard (summarized in Fisher et al. 2007) reported on a sample that spans 200 years. The Albany sample was, at the time it was analyzed, the largest intestinal parasite sample from urban contexts. Albany began construction on a sewer system in 1850, and advertisements for privy cleaning services were still present in the 1870s (Fisher et al. 2007: 177). Even though those advertisements indicate that privies remained in use following the sewer system construction, a law in 1872 that forbade dumping garbage and debris in privies might have impacted their levels of contamination. Unlike the study of the Five Points area, the study from Albany spanned a large time segment and a number of social classes.

Reinhard found a number of things about trends in parasite infestation in Albany. Roundworms seem to have been a major problem since the seventeenth century. "Five different human parasites were identified in the archaeological samples collected from Albany. They include the *Ascaris* (roundworm), *Trichuris* (whipworm), *Taenia* (tapeworm), *Hymenolepiasis nana* (dwarf tapeworm), and the first archaeological observation of the parasite *Macracanthorhynchus hirudinaceus*" (Fisher et al. 2007: 187). Rapid population growth is associated with increased numbers of parasite eggs. There is a general decline in parasite eggs after 1830 which seems to be associated with a shift in the methods of privy construction. "The earlier wooden barrels in the ground were replaced with wooden box vaults in the early-19th century, which were augmented later by the use of stone-lined vaults. This trend reflects the effort to control seepage of waste from the privies into the surrounding soil" (Fisher et al. 2007: 190).

Privies were not just utilized in urban contexts, despite the focus in this chapter thus far. However, the sanitation problems they caused were visibly apparent in urban settings in a way that they remained visibly unnoticed (at least initially) in rural contexts. They were, of course, fairly universal buildings for relieving oneself throughout America after the seventeenth century. In the last quarter of the nineteenth century, urban sanitation campaigns largely eradicated the use of privies in the larger urban centers as centralized sewage systems allowed for adequate sewage disposal.

However, their use endured far longer in rural contexts well into the twentieth century. The year 1909 was a major turning point in public health connected to human waste disposal. In that year, John D. Rockefeller formed the Rockefeller Sanitary Commission with the explicit duty of combating hookworm disease, which was rampant in the largely rural southern states of America. Numerous public health pamphlets and articles stressed the importance of the sanitary privy in preventing hookworm, which is fundamentally linked to fecal contamination (see Lay 1910 for a discussion of the sanitary privy). That design began as the Rochdale Pail System in the last quarter of the nineteenth century and was improved upon slightly by the Sanitary Privy in the early 1900s. In either case, the filled pails were intended to be taken away from the residence and emptied.

Privies still exist today, mostly in rural places, although in rest areas along highways and in parks one still encounters numerous privies, albeit somewhat upgraded in design with contained waste receptacles. Privy use can still extend rather close to cities. In 1996, for instance, there were 50,000 homes without indoor plumbing in the greater Research Triangle area of North Carolina and at that time, the article reports, "North Carolina remains one of the top outhouse states in the nation" (Stohler 1996).

Sanitary Reform

Water and Sewage

> Complaint is made that your family throws swill teagrounds etc. into the cesspool in your backyard and the same has clogged the drain and will have to be cleaned out which our Mr. Crawford will attend to, but you must stop throwing such stuff into the drain and not have it [happen] again, and use your swill bucket for such things. Also you had a dead cat in your ash barrel last Friday which had lain so long that it was maggatey. You must be more cleanly, and not have so much litter about your premises, as it will breed disease and *can't be allowed*. (letter dated September 3, 1889, to a tenant at Boott Mills, unit 54

[Boott Cotton Mills Corporation 1889–1891, 290] cited in Mrozowski et al. 1989: 304)

The mid- to late nineteenth century saw a much increased devotion to sanitation. While there is no one instigating factor, a number of things contributed to the attention to cleanliness. Sanitation and disinfection became evident targets of reform during the Civil War. Especially important for bringing sanitation to the attention of many during the war was the development of the United States Sanitary Commission, which was established in 1861. After the war, attention to sanitation continued and major targets were cities and the dwellings within them, particularly with regard to human waste, refuse, and ventilation. As indicated in the Boott Cotton Mills letter above, disposal of garbage was among many items of increased attention with regard to hygiene.

There was an increased value during the sanitary reform placed on proper light and ventilation in creating a healthy environment and preventing contagion. An important contribution was David Boswell Reid's *Ventilation in American Dwellings* (1858). Crowding was another issue that some saw as a major component of health. Quite simply, infectious disease and poor hygiene seemed to be worse in the crowded tenements of the poor.

Human waste disposal during the sanitary reform period continued to be less than ideal. Everyone agreed that privies were fine in rural settings, but they were immense environmental hazards in crowded cities. They simply had to give way to other forms of toilet mechanics. Several innovations were attempted over the years, but attention was often directed toward moving sewage along with water, since drainage was already an established concept. Water closets (rooms with flush toilets) were one such innovation, but the water to utilize them was often still in short supply.

Consequently, there were some water closets, but their expense was out of reach for many, and there wasn't really an adequate supply of water until after the mid-nineteenth century to service them. Thus, privies were the primary means of providing a toilet until the last half of the nineteenth century in major cities. Water supply was a major barrier to toilet reform. Two major issues centered on water: adequate supply for purposes beyond consumption, and where to send wastewater once it was soiled.

The opening of the Croton Aqueduct in 1842 began to change the water supply issues in New York, and water consumption increased generally. Another innovation was the availability of piped-in water. The opening of the Croton viaduct was quickly followed in lower Manhattan by pipes being laid, which made piped-in water available for many people by 1850. Plumbing reached most middle-class homes in urban centers across America, as well as in some working-class homes, by 1860 (Green 1986: 108).

With an adequate supply of water, many more people turned to water closets, but there remained the problem of where the sewage was to go. As water closets came into vogue, the densely populated City of New York saw increased sewage problems, as most sewers were designed to handle runoff and drainage, not the increased sewage from private households. To make things worse, the old sewage system there was outdated and undermaintained.

There was a resistance to building substantial underground sewer systems because sewers had generally been built to address specific groundwater drainage problems; they usually did not have enough slope to drain sewage properly. "Moreover, careless street cleaning methods and the tendency of the public to throw anything and everything into the streets, including dead animals, rapidly clogged up the sewers. Since the latter had no trapping devices, the odor from their putrefying contents, particularly during the summer months, escaped from the catch basins and made life almost unbearable for nearby residents" (Duffy 1968: 406). Nonetheless, in 1844, residents in New York were allowed to hook water closets to the sewer system, inadequate as it was. It was not until between 1847 and 1857 when some parts of New York received adequate sewers.

To add to the sewage problems, water closets were increasingly hooked to cesspools which were inadequate to handle the volume of water and waste. With an adequate supply of water provided by the Croton viaduct, cisterns became less necessary as freshwater containment receptacles. Punching holes into the bottom made them ideal for becoming cesspools and receiving sewage. The cesspools soon overflowed, however, contaminating the water in gutters and storm drains. A number of former rainwater cisterns were converted into cesspools once Croton provided water, and the problems created by the practice were noted by Dr. John Griscom in his marvelous document *The Sanitary Condition of the Laboring Population*:

> Since the introduction of the Croton, the rain water cisterns being useless, the bottoms of them have in many instances been taken out, and they have been converted into cispools, into which refuse matter of the houses is thrown. Great trouble is thus saved to families and domestics, but it needs no prophetic vision to perceive, that an

immense mass of offensive materials, will thus soon be collected, its decomposition polluting the air, in the immediate precincts of our chambers and sitting rooms, and generating an amount of miasmatic effluvia, incalculably great and injurious. Discharge all the contents of our sinks and cispools, through sewers into the rivers, and we will avoid two of the most powerful causes of sickness and early death. (Griscom 1845: 52)

Two of the cisterns at the Sullivan Street site exhibited exactly that conversion—their bottoms had been knocked out.

The availability of increased access to water, now piped into many urban homes, did not solve all of the water problems. Fresh water for consumption remained a problem in New York. One stimulus to centralized water systems was the emergence of frequent cholera epidemics. Cholera visited New York in 1832 and again in 1849. It was not the only stimulus though; New York, like most cities, always struggled in the early nineteenth century with providing clean water for consumption and disposal of refuse and waste. Two things began to change the water and sewer situation during the next decade: a campaign for public awareness of the sanitation issues by the newspapers, and rapid advances in sewer and water supply designs by British engineers in London.

After the British experienced their own cholera epidemics in 1849 and 1854, Dr. John Snow made the connection between water contamination and cholera, particularly as linked to sewage in the water supply. He noted that the most severe outbreaks of cholera tended to be in very localized areas of London, usually inhabited by the poorer segments of society. In September of 1854, a particularly serious cholera outbreak occurred in Soho, and Snow suspected the water pump on Broad Street (now Broadwick Street), was linked to the infections.

Snow mapped the cases in the area, which all centered on the Broad Street pump, and upon further investigation found that many of those not ill with cholera worked in the local brewery and didn't consume the well water. After Snow drew some of the water into a vessel and let it stand for a couple of days, it turned opaque and foul-smelling. With no further evidence than that, he nonetheless persuaded officials to remove the pump handle. Within a few weeks the outbreak subsided.

In 1852, London passed the Metropolis Water Act prohibiting water companies from obtaining their water from the Thames River, and in the early 1900s the private companies were nationalized. New York made its own water supply improvements, no doubt stimulated by success in London, and the city saw immense growth in extent and in design of the underground sewer system between 1849 and 1860. Water quality, however, remained somewhat of an issue.

While the growth of underground sewers was taking place, there remained numerous privies in the poorer tenements, and runoff and seepage could easily contaminate drinking water. Methods of filtering water became extremely popular after 1870, with both portable filters that serviced individual households and those which serviced buildings. The larger building-service models were usually hooked right up to the water supply and were quite expensive, so most people relied on filters they could pour water through.

Two innovations were designed during the second half of the nineteenth century to alleviate the problems of water-based toilet systems and potable water. The earth closet, or commode, was a chamber with a seat; the deposits emptied into a vessel containing earth (Figure 7.1). The seat opening had a cover and a tank at the back of the apparatus held extra dry earth. Earth closets were said to prevent cholera from entering the water system, to waste no good fertilizer material, and to reduce the possibility of sewer gas buildup.

> The earth-closet is an invention which relieves the most disagreeable item in domestic labor, and prevents the disagreeable and unhealthful effluvium which is almost inevitable in all family residences. The general principle of construction is somewhat like that of a water-closet, except that in place of water is used dried earth. The resulting compost is without disagreeable odor, and is the richest species of manure. The expense of its construction and use is no greater than that of the common water-closet; indeed, when the outlays for plumber's work, the almost inevitable troubles and disorders of water-pipes in a house, and the construction or use of water-works are considered, the earth-closet is in itself much cheaper, besides being an accumulator of valuable matter. (Beecher and Stowe 1971 [1869]: 403)

The parlor commode appeared about 1900 and was designed to alleviate those odors that did emerge from commodes by venting the commode through a stovepipe into the wood stove. Their popularity was limited, partly because the system actually didn't work that well, but largely because by 1900 advances in plumbing reached a point where water-based sewage disposal was a fully operational system.

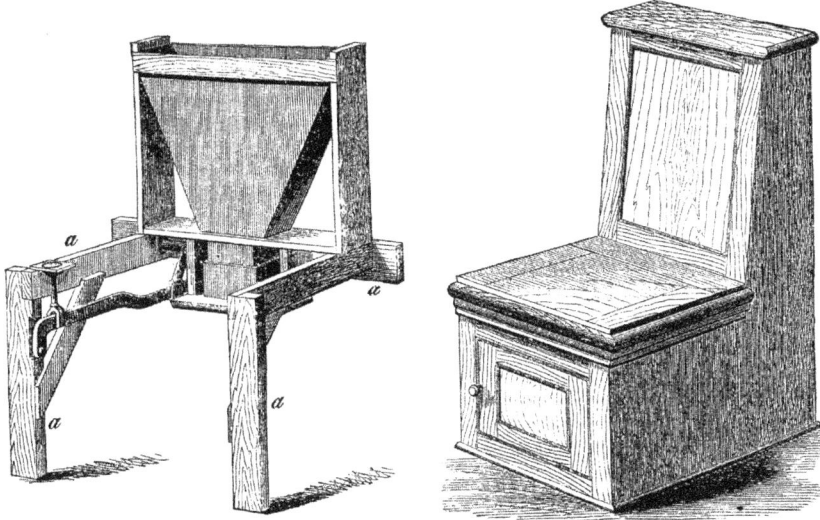

Figure 7.1. Design for an earth closet (*left*) to sit within a commode (*right*). Adapted from Beecher and Stowe 1971 (originally published 1869), Figures 67 and 69.

Hygiene and the Home

America became completely focused on healthy living through sanitation after 1850, especially after the acceptance of the germ theory of disease following 1875 or so.

Sanitary reform after 1875 focused heavily on the home. *Household Manual of Domestic Hygiene, Food and Diet*, by Kellogg (1882); *Our Homes* (Murphy 1883); *Principles of Domestic Science* (Beecher and Stowe 1971 [1869]); and *Godey's Lady's Book* (periodical) all provided guidance for what makes a clean and healthy domicile.

Every household furnishing and surface was subject to consideration and potential reformation. Carpets and window curtains, books, old wooden floors, were all seen as potential dust magnets. Reform-style houses in America called "Eastlake Houses" were built with wood floors to minimize dust and they were usually furnished with simple furniture. There were lots of windows in Eastlake houses for ventilation and light. Various floor sweepers were manufactured to handle dust and dirt—one of the best known was made by the Bissell Carpet Sweeper Company in Grand Rapids, Michigan.

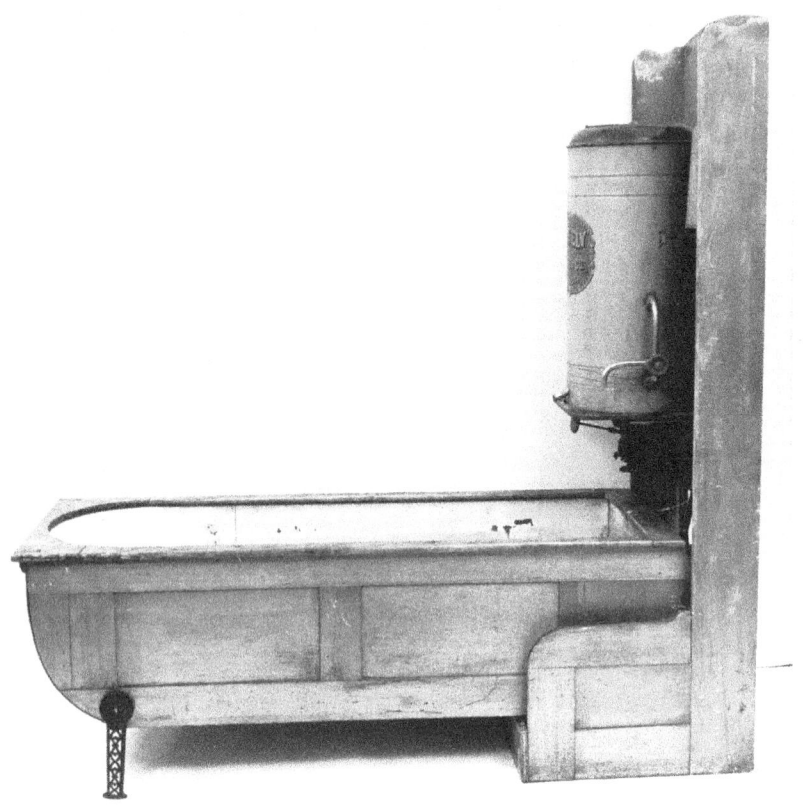

Figure 7.2. Moseley folding bathtub, circa 1880–1900. Used by permission of National Museum of American History. ID number 1977.1217.13, catalog number 1977.1217.13, accession number 1977.1217, Credit Line Crane Company. Division of Cultural and Community Life, National Museum of American History, Smithsonian Institution.

The second half of the nineteenth century was a time of numerous cases of consumption (TB), and ventilation was on everyone's mind. Sleeping quarters were especially subject to sanitary reform, and the perfect bedroom was well ventilated, free of carpeting, had closets for clothing, and pillows of an alternative filling to feathers, such as straw or seagrass (Green 1986: 125). Even beds were under scrutiny in the reform. Feather beds were denounced by many, and a rather loud voice among the detractors was that of John Harvey Kellogg, who thought them very unhealthy because they suffer from "slow decomposition. . . . thus evolving foul and poisonous gases" (cited in Green 1986: 123). Tied spring mattresses had been manufactured since the 1830s and served as the replacement for the feather mattress.

Personal hygiene received a lot of attention coincident with the microscope enabling the examination of microorganisms that were linked to specific diseases. From parasites on the skin to clogged pores, daily bathing became a national theme: "Every family, rich and poor, ought to have a bathing machine, improperly called a tub. It is easy of construction, and very simple, being in shape like a child's cradle without rockers, about six feet in length, and of width sufficiently easy to admit the body, with a hole in the bottom near the foot, to let the water pass off after being used" (Gunn 1830: 161).

Hot water, bathtubs, soaps, and bathing gear began to appear in the typical American household. The goal of every middle- and wealthy-class American was to have a permanent, stationary tub located in a separate toilet room. If one could not afford a permanent, stationary bathtub, the options included portable washstands and the Universal Bath. The latter was essentially a rubberized sheet with a wooden rim that was supported by a chair on each end. Alternatively, if one did have adequate room, there was the Moseley folding bathtub which dropped down and had a water-heating tank, and then folded back into a luxurious wooden cabinet (Figure 7.2).

* * *

Prior to the Civil War, recognition that medical care in America was foundering was widespread. Teetering on the brink of complete collapse, with regard both to institutional failures and distrust of the general public, the Civil War instigated reform. With the termination of the war, Americans were ready to effect other changes toward better health and well-being. Hygiene became a major focus of reform. Advances in water supply, sewage systems, and home cleanliness all enabled a reduction of health and wellness issues related to hygiene. Behind the scenes, for many, were advances in the recognition of disease-causing agents. Pasteur, Lister, and others, familiar names now, were making discoveries that settled once and for all where diseases come from and what causes them.

8

Hospital Reformation and Redirection

> Even in the best run hospitals, chronically straitened budgets dictated that patients would find no frills or luxuries. Early in the nineteenth century especially, crowded rooms and eighteenth-century sensibilities meant that operations would ordinarily be performed in the common ward; similarly, patients might die and be placed in coffins within sight and smell of the surviving patients.
>
> (Rosenberg 1987: 31)

By 1850, half a century of declining funds for hospitals left the institutional care of the infirm insufficient for most people. As Rosenberg points out, there was simply not sufficient funding to maintain any good standard of care. It was not only funding that was lacking, however. It was the lack of support from those who found medical practitioners suspect. It was the changing demography and economy of America. It was disagreement among physicians and scientists about the causative factors of illness. The Civil War brought about many needed reforms for institutional care, but there was more to be done.

The post–Civil War health reformation was not limited to urban infrastructure and domestic space. Alongside the domestic reform movement were changes in the sanitation of hospitals. Hospital design in the form of the pavilion hospital created cleaner, more healthy conditions, but also there was a growing realization that some health and wellness conditions required long-term, specialized care. The underlying purpose of institutional care was directed at special needs—tuberculosis and mental health—with a new approach of social and environmental healing. In the course of all of these changes, the discovery of microorganisms demonstrated the undeniable facts regarding the causative agents of disease and ushered in the germ theory of disease. It was no small contribution in the reformation of late-nineteenth-century health and wellness.

Hospital Reform

Hygiene was a central part of hospital reform, and the cleaning, airing, and sterilizing of patient spaces, especially those that had recently housed infectious patients, became a primary concern. A name almost synonymous with hospital hygiene reform is that of Florence Nightingale. Her emphasis on an ordered and clean environment in Britain's military hospitals during the Crimean War (between 1854 and 1856) was an impetus for reform on both sides of the Atlantic (Rosenberg 1987: 135). It came at a propitious time as America was about to enter its own period of intense military hospitals with the Civil War (1861–1865; see Chapter 6).

Coincident with the hospital reform movement was a debate about the origin of hospital infections. The majority of hospital workers, Nightingale included, believed that the origin of infections was tied to the atmosphere. Most people in the first half of the nineteenth century thought atmospheric gases were a primary cause of infection; therefore, placing patients into tight, overcrowded spaces increased the risk of contracting diseases. Quite simply, the more people that were crowded into small spaces and who shared the same air, and the more filth was present in those spaces, the more frequently people became infected.

Consequently, new policies were implemented to combat infections acquired in hospitals: avoid overcrowding, enforce cleanliness, and promote ventilation. These new policies also affected hospital design as new hospitals were planned during the hospital building boom of the late 1860s and 1870s (Rosenberg 1987: 137). A principal consideration when siting a new hospital was that it be far away from the city center, preferably in an area located near open fields and a body of water from which cleansing air could flow easily through the building. These new guidelines were implemented within the context of the pavilion hospital, a plan that emphasized hospitals with long wings and rooms with lots of windows running parallel down the long axis of the wings. The entire design was made so as to maximize air flow and sunlight, and was partially made in response to the prevailing theories that stressed atmospheric gases (miasmas) as the major cause of disease.

There was growing scientific evidence, however, that the actual causative factors of disease were not atmospheric gases but physical agents of infection (Billings 1875a: 33). Although a notion of particulate, disease-causing matter was present at least as far back as Greek scholars Thucydides and

Galen, supportive scientific evidence really began to accumulate in the early 1860s. It was the laboratory research of Louis Pasteur in the 1860s and then Robert Koch in the following decades that provided the scientific proof for germ theory.

Proving the germ theory of disease was the crowning achievement of the French scientist Louis Pasteur. He was not the first to propose that diseases were caused by microscopic organisms, and the view was controversial in the nineteenth century, as it opposed the accepted theory of "spontaneous generation." At that time, Pasteur had demonstrated the growth of microorganisms in nutrient broth and that sealing the broth from the atmosphere could prevent their growth. Not only did Pasteur discover that decomposition was caused by microbes, but he discovered that heat could kill microbes; thus, the credit to his name—*pasteurization,* appropriately first used for wine.

Pasteur's work inspired Joseph Lister, who campaigned for decontamination of hospital spaces using carbolic acid in the mid-1860s. If decomposition could be caused by microorganisms, Lister reasoned, the same principle could be applied to wounds and surgical incisions. Antiseptic surgery is generally attributed to Lister, and a credit is due also to his namesake product, *Listerine.* By the early 1870s, Pasteur's and Lister's ideas were being widely discussed in scientific journals and undoubtedly influenced John Shaw Billings, the former Surgeon General of the Union Army, who produced several treatises on military hygiene (Billings 1870, 1875a, 1875b).

Billings was an insightful doctor who continued to adjust his perspectives on hygiene given the most recent scientific discussions. His perspective on contamination, combined with his appreciation of germ theory, put him ahead of many of his contemporaries:

> The air in a hospital ward is made impure and harmful in two very different ways.
>
> First, it is contaminated with gases derived from the lungs and bodies of the patients, from the decompositions of their secretions and excretia, and from the products of combustion. These gases are carbonic oxide, and carbonic acid, sulphuretted and phosphuretted hydrogen, and ammonia and its compounds and substitute products. . . .
>
> The second kind of contamination in a hospital consists of minute particles of solid or semi-solid matter, derived directly or indirectly from the bodies of the patients, of which they once formed a part.

Some of these particles, if placed in contact with a living surface, as of the mouth or lungs, or of a wound, will either grow and reproduce themselves, or they will change the mode of action of the part with which they come in contact, or they may do both, and in either event will affect the blood, and weaken or alter the natural process of life; in other words, they will cause or aggravate disease.

It is to these particles, known as disease germs, contagia, microzymes, micrococci, bioplasm, germinal matter, etc., according to the different theories which are held as to their nature and mode of action, that are supposed to be due the majority, if not all, of the contagious and infectious diseases, including those specially prevalent in hospitals and referred to in the term "Hospitalism." . . .

Whatever may be the opinions held as to the nature of these diseased germs, and their mode of origin and propagation, they are what we have to fear and to provide against in the construction of a hospital. They are on and in the dressings, the sponges, the instruments and apparatus, the bedding and clothing of the patients, the persons and clothing of the physicians and attendants. (Billings 1875b: 33–34)

Billing's influence would go far beyond the military. He was one of the consultants for the construction of Johns Hopkins Hospital (Billings 1875a), and he included many of the innovations he had witnessed for army medical facilities. The familiar pavilion plan characterized the general plan for Johns Hopkins Hospital, with separate surgical pavilions, kitchens and laundry, free patient rooms, and private patient rooms (Figure 6.1). Ventilation was provided by a combination of ridge ventilation and foul air ducts (see Billings 1875a for a full description of how the ventilation system worked).

By the end of the 1880s the miasma theory was struggling to compete with the germ theory of disease. Eventually, a "golden era" of bacteriology ensued, during which the germ theory of disease quickly led to the identification of the actual organisms that cause many diseases. The debate about contagion versus environment was somewhat put to rest with Robert Koch's discoveries of the tuberculosis and cholera organisms in 1882 and 1883.

Sterilization

The logical outcome of the acceptance of germ theory was to devise a way to prevent contamination through the eradication of germs. Although Lister had started the process through chemical disinfection in the mid-nineteenth century, heat and water became the major ways to thoroughly clean items after 1875. Pasteur's student and collaborator, Charles Chamberland, developed the first pressure steam sterilizer, or autoclave, in 1876. The same year John Tyndall, an English physicist, discovered heat-resistant bacteria.

It was Koch and his associates who discovered that steam and hot air would serve for sterilization in 1881, and they developed the first nonpressure flowing steam sterilizer. In 1881 as well, sterilization by boiling was introduced into medical practice and everything used during an operation, including linens, dressings, and gowns, was boiled. Boiling was not universally accepted for some years though, and some surgeons still believed Lister's method was adequate.

By the early 1900s, sterilization was a standard practice and most medical facilities had some sort of sterilization equipment. In order to keep instruments and other materials sterile, containers were developed to house the sterile materials until further use. Sterilization remained the standard practice until the 1960s when disposable instruments and other materials used in medical settings were developed. Disposable medical supplies, unfortunately, are a problem with regard to proper disposal and their use is currently debated in medical literature (for example, Arnold 2009; Olson 2009).

Special Facilities, Special Needs

> When we consider the rapid advances made by the world in every branch of social improvement, we cannot too strongly stigmatize the manner in which the inmates [in] some of public institutions are treated—especially the indigent mentally ill—for whom it would seem there is not a single gleam of commiseration or charity to break the horrid gloom in which their lives are shrouded. It cannot be denied that the practice which prevails in many of the counties of herding the mentally ill in jails or almshouses, instead of sending them to a proper asylum, where their shattered minds would be brought nearer to the fountain care, is a crime against God, against society, and against individuals; a shame to our civilization and a blot on our age. (Chancellor 1877: 11)

There was not any one reason that special facilities paved the way for special care. Rather it was a combination of things: the collapse of the hospital system, the failure of the almshouse, a recognition that health-care institutions should have more selective and categorical terms than "illness." Alongside those selective categories of different types of illnesses was a burgeoning recognition that different approaches and facilities were required for some health and well-being issues. As Chancellor espouses, special facilities were not simply institutions that placed the poor away from middle- and upper-class society, as were almshouses; they were designed to provide care for specific health problems that usually required long-term care. As such, they generally had a caring, benign, and humane approach in both staff and building design, at least for a while, that almshouses lacked.

Asylums for the Mentally Ill

Institutional care of the mentally ill in early colonial America began in the late seventeenth and eighteenth centuries, although the earliest institutions were really almshouses that accepted the mentally ill (Grob 1973: 13). General hospitals initially provided care for the mentally ill and mentally unbalanced, but by the 1820s there was increasing social pressure to separate those physically ill from those termed "lunatics" or "mentally ill." As well, the dramatic population growth that was occurring at that time saw a proportionate increase in the mentally ill, and they were often more visible in urban spaces. They frankly made the general population nervous and uneasy.

The first hospital in America was the Pennsylvania Hospital, which accepted its first patients in 1752. Throughout the eighteenth century, the Pennsylvania Hospital cared for patients who were mentally ill, but the number of mentally ill patients was never large: 18 between 1752 and 1754, 34 by 1787 (Grob 1994: 19). Patients were frequently held in confined spaces. For instance, in the Pennsylvania Hospital, cells were constructed in the basement, and around the outside wall ran a moat. The public could stand on the far side of that moat and watch the patients through their windows (Thompson and Goldin 1975: 76).

In those early institutions that housed the mentally ill, restraint by either leather or iron straps for prolonged periods was common. It was used to "quiet" the patient. Dr. Benjamin Rush, one of the doctors at the Pennsylvania Hospital, developed a tranquilizer chair which held the patient restrained at the hands, arms, legs, and chest while restricting vision to a limited forward area (Figure 8.1).

Mental asylums, also known as mental hospitals, and even later as state hospitals, had their roots in eighteenth-century hospitals. The first hospital

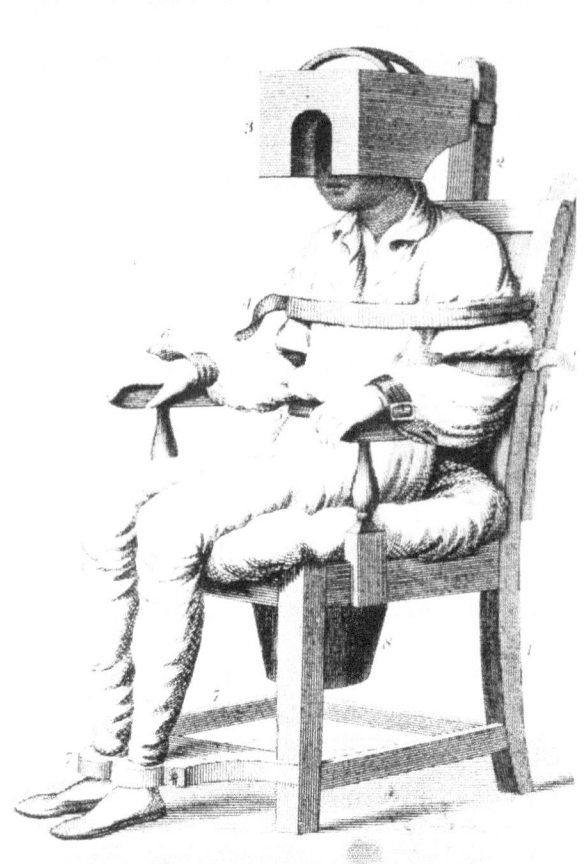

Figure 8.1. Tranquilizer chair of Benjamin Rush. Wood engraving, National Library of Medicine, Unique ID: 101436673 (see catalog record), NLM Image ID: A013394.

specifically designed for the care and treatment of the mentally ill was the Public Hospital for the Persons of Mentally Ill and Disordered Minds which opened in 1773 in Williamsburg, Virginia. During the earliest years of that hospital, chemical and physical treatments "drained the system of harmful fluids, reduced inflammation, and refocused the patient's attention" (Zwelling 1985: 15). There were bleedings, purgings, immersion in hot or cold water, blistering, and as early as 1793, electrical shock in the form of electrostatic shock via an electrostatic generator (Zwelling 1985: 15). Massachusetts General Hospital opened a separate hospital in 1818 for psychiatric care, and Pennsylvania Hospital opened a second hospital, the Pennsylvania Hospital for the Insane, in 1841. By the next decade, most private hospitals placed mental illness as a condition ineligible for admission.

It was about the same time, the mid-1800s, that the treatment of the mentally ill turned from an approach of incarceration to one of a "moral treatment." One of the very influential psychiatrists at the time, Thomas Story Kirkbride, used his medical and administrative experience as the head of Pennsylvania Hospital for the Mentally Ill to advocate a moral and environmental approach to mental illness. It was one borrowed from late eighteenth century England which emphasized several facets of creating an environment of health and wellness (Tomes 2001). Moral treatment, as practiced by Kirkbride and others, avoided restraints, incarceration, or drug intervention. Rather, healing and wellness were facilitated through social interaction, kindness, and the restorative powers of a connection with the natural world to create a "therapeutic landscape."

Kirkbride's book on asylum design was widely used and emphasized the healing importance of hospital buildings and grounds (Kirkbride 1854). The "Kirkbride plan," as it became known, stressed that common spaces inside were immense and numerous, while individual rooms were kept small, about 9 by 8 feet. Abundant sunlight and good ventilation were vital to the healing process; every patient's room had a window with a view to the outside and ventilation ducts. Air was drawn from outside and circulated through immense tunnels, up into the building, and out through large porticos on top of the building which created updrafts.

The grounds outside were immense, often with ponds, forests, open grassland, numerous benches, and recreation areas, much like large parks. Parts of the Kirkbride plan were uniquely centered on the social aspects of asylum space, but it is important to recognize that the actual structure of the building, oriented horizontally rather than vertically, and the emphasis on ventilation and sunlight, were simply part of the pavilion hospital plan developed during the Civil War.

A perfect example of the Kirkbride plan is the Traverse City State Hospital (formerly the Northern Michigan Asylum). Located outside of town, as many pavilion hospitals following the Kirkbride plan were, it looked out over Grand Traverse Bay. Begun in April of 1883, construction took fewer than three years to complete, and by November of 1885, it received its first patients. The main structure, Building 50, was planned as a large structure—almost one quarter mile long, over 300,000 square feet, and over 70 feet tall at the roof ridge (Figure 8.2).

Over 8 million bricks were brought from the local brickyard at Cedar Lake to construct Building 50. It included several distinct wards for men and women (separately), as well as a chapel, library, and kitchen/dining

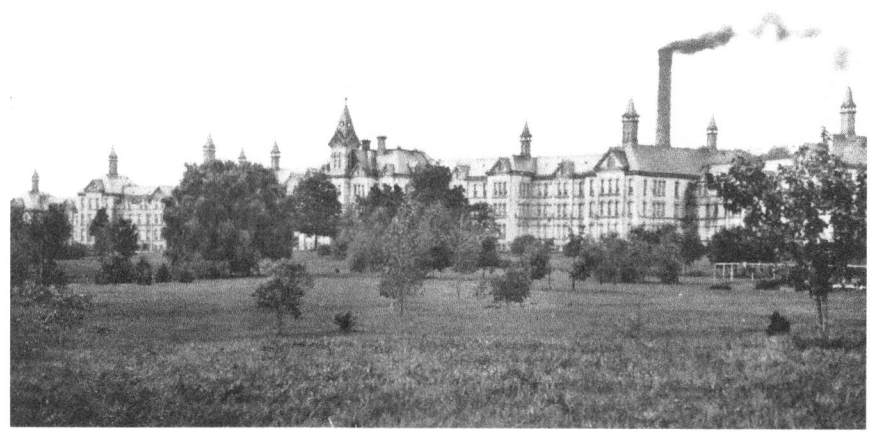

Figure 8.2. Northern Michigan Asylum, Building 50, 1909. Image courtesy of the Local History Collection, Traverse Area District Library.

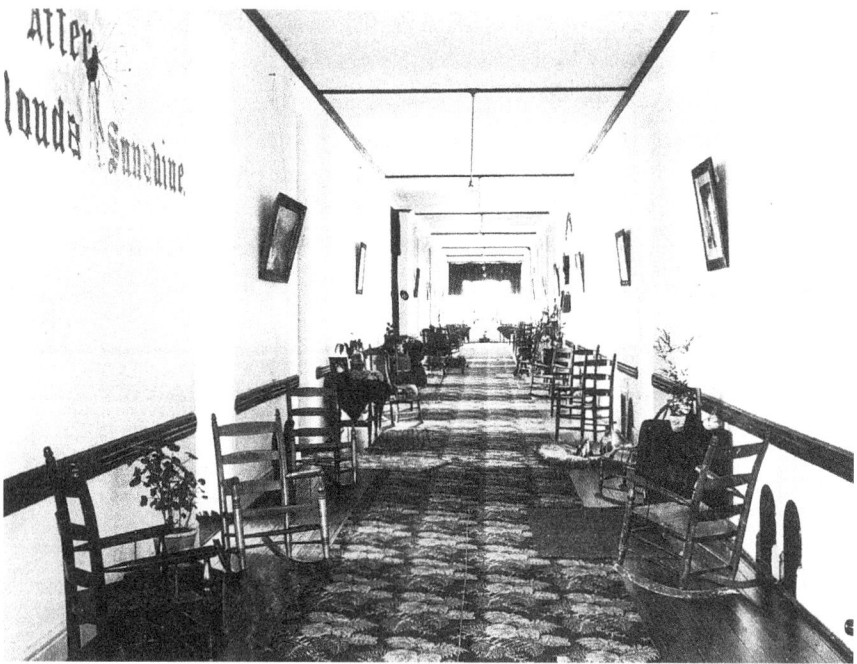

Figure 8.3. Northern Michigan Asylum Men's Ward sitting area. Image courtesy of the Local History Collection, Traverse Area District Library.

areas with central heat and electric lights (Figure 8.3). The chapel served additionally as a concert and dance hall. The four-sided tower at the top center of Building 50 with the semicircular slatted areas is the ventilation tower.

A state-of-the-art ventilation system was designed for the Northern Michigan Asylum which utilized large fans to force air through underground tunnels into the basement, and from there up flues into the various parts of the building. The ventilation system thus worked like a chimney, with the air moving through ducts within the attic and exiting through the ventilation tower or "spire," much in the same way as Billings ridge vents.

At the time of its completion, the Northern Michigan Asylum served 39 counties, including all of the Upper Peninsula, and almost immediately there was demand for additional patient rooms. Starting in the 1890s, stand-alone cottages were constructed to serve the increasing patient population (Figure 8.4). The cottages were segregated in the same way as Building 50—cottages to the south which were even-numbered were for the men, and the cottages to the north and odd-numbered were for the women.

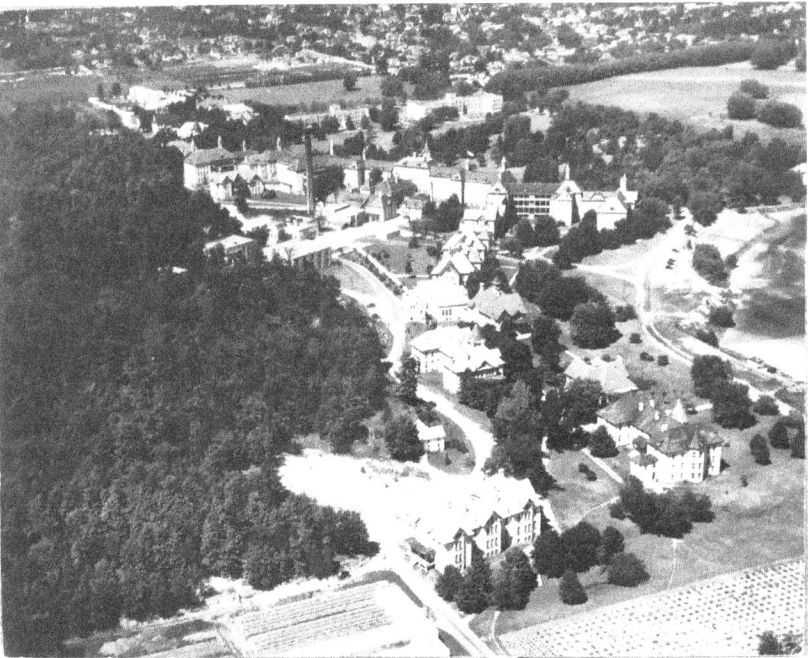

Figure 8.4. Aerial View, Northern Michigan Asylum, Building 50 (*top*) and surrounding cottages (*bottom*). Image courtesy of the Michigan History Center, Archives of Michigan.

Cottages also provided spaces to separate patients from the larger population based on severity of condition, age, or illness. For example, Cottage 25 was a tuberculosis ward, Cottage 29 a geriatric ward, and Cottage 27 an epileptic ward (Johnson 2001: 30–31).

Traverse City State Hospital included some 60 buildings at its height of operations that consisted of specialized cottages for women and men, children, tuberculosis patients, and the elderly. The entire hospital operation housed 2,200 people in the 1920s, a fairly large population since the population of Traverse City was only 6,000; patients were not included in the census counts since they were mostly from other counties (Steele and Hains 2001: 16). There were a number of supporting operations that included administrative offices, carriage barns, greenhouse, powerhouse, laundry, water tower, carpentry and furniture repair shop, fire station, bakery, icehouse and meat storage house, nurse's training area, staff housing, fruit and vegetable warehouse, rag- and soap-house, machine and electrical shop, TV repair shop, and specialized care facilities (for example, children's hospital, geriatric hospital, tuberculosis hospital, and residence hall; Decker 2010; Johnson 2001).

Founding Medical Superintendent Dr. James Munson made an effort to ensure that patients felt at home rather than trapped in an unfamiliar place. Use of physical restraints was forbidden, except for the most extreme patient situations. Meals at the hospital were served in dining rooms on fine china glazed with the state seal atop white linen tablecloths (Figure 8.5). Fresh flowers and plants decorated dining tables and resting areas.

After closing in 1989, like so many government structures, the buildings and grounds fell into neglect. In 1993, the property was transferred from the State of Michigan to the Grand Traverse Commons Redevelopment Corporation. Some buildings were turned into government offices, and others were demolished. In 2000 the Minervini Group began negotiating with the Grand Traverse Commons Redevelopment Corporation and secured an agreement to renovate the historic buildings. The buildings are slowly being remodeled and restored as the Village at Grand Traverse Commons. Building 50 now houses numerous restaurants and shops as well as residential apartments. There are several excellent histories and photographic essays on Traverse City Hospital (Decker 2010; Johnson 2001; Miller 2005; Steele and Hains 2001) and tours of the property operate during the summer.

Unfortunately, "beautiful therapy" did not last as an approach to mental health care. It was followed by drug therapy, lobotomy, and electric shock therapy. The golden age of treating mental health from a perspective of

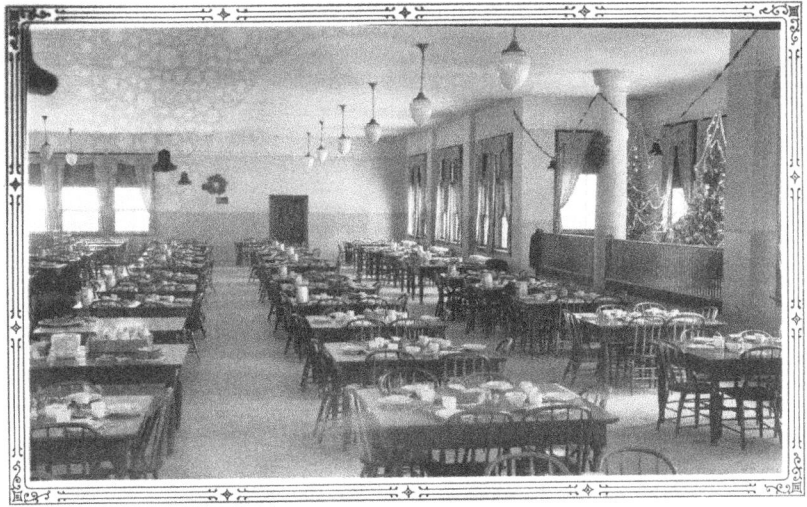

Figure 8.5. One of the men's dining rooms at the Traverse City State Hospital showing their Christmas tree, December 25, 1935. Image courtesy of the Michigan History Center, Archives of Michigan.

gentle healing through social interaction, and ample light and ventilation, gave way to rooms with bars and portions of buildings with locked doors. "Healing walks in the sunshine" and fresh air were replaced with sedation, physical restraints, electric shock—all familiar through Ken Kesey's depiction of an asylum in *One Flew Over the Cuckoo's Nest* (Kesey 1970), or in Sylvia Plath's *The Bell Jar* (Plath 1971).

> Through the slits of my eyes, which I didn't dare open too far, lest the full view strike me dead, I saw the high bed with its white, drumtight sheet, and the machine behind the bed, and the masked person—I couldn't tell whether it was a man or a woman—behind the machine, and other masked people flanking the bed on both sides.
> Miss Huey helped me climb up and lie down on my back.
> "Talk to me," I said.
> Miss Huey began to talk in a low, soothing voice, smoothing the salve on my temples and fitting the small electric buttons on either side of my head. "You'll be perfectly all right, you won't feel a thing, just bite down . . ." And she set something on my tongue and in a panic I bit down, and darkness wiped me out like chalk on a blackboard (Sylvia Plath, *The Bell Jar*, 1971: 175).

Tuberculosis Sanatoria

> To Cure Sometimes, to Relieve Often, to Comfort Always.
> (from a plaque at Saranac Lake)

Tuberculosis (TB) is caused by a rod-shaped bacterium known as a spirochete. It was Robert Koch who in 1882 isolated the cause of tuberculosis, and his discovery is often said to have initiated a public health campaign, although tuberculosis sanatoria have historical roots going back at least to the sixteenth century in Europe (Dubos and Dubos 1996; Roberts and Buikstra 2003). Tuberculosis is a disease of malnutrition, poverty, and crowded, poorly ventilated domiciles. In the United States, it was a disease that in the nineteenth century killed one in five people, although it impacted urban dwellers especially hard with a mortality rate of 300 per 100,000 persons (Cole 1935: 8; Roberts and Buikstra 2003: 236). Four hundred TB patients died per day of the disease in 1907 (Gallos 1985: 16).

The first four American hospitals for tuberculosis patients, all free, were established in Boston and Philadelphia between 1857 and 1876. A fifth private sanatorium was established in 1875 by Dr. Joseph Gleizmann in Asheville, North Carolina (Roberts and Buikstra 2003). Creation of TB sanatoria in America followed at a rapid pace. In 1904, 115 facilities (about 8,000 beds) were operating, a number that reached 839 institutions (more than 136,000 beds) in 1953 (Daniel 1997; Murray et al. 2015). They would be, until drug therapy, the primary way to cure the disease.

Despite these earlier sanatoria, however, the popularity of sanatorium treatment in America is usually credited to Dr. Edward Livingston Trudeau who began his facility at Saranac Lake, New York, with the construction of the cure cottage "Little Red" in 1885, only three years after Robert Koch discovered the pathogen (bacillus) that causes tuberculosis. A tuberculosis patient himself, Dr. Trudeau found that on repeated visits to the highlands of Saranac Lake, far north of New York City, his health improved.

Nestled into the Adirondack Mountains, Saranac Lake has many months per year of cold, mountain air. It was Trudeau's experiments in outdoor living and its effect on tuberculosis recovery that would popularize lifestyle change as a cure for tuberculosis. His prescribed treatment was one of healthy living, abundant rest, fresh air (cold, fresh air was preferable), and when possible, light exercise. Nutritious food was emphasized, as was abstinence from alcohol.

Dr. Trudeau designed his facilities at Saranac Lake to accommodate the working class who had less money—the standard rate for everyone was five

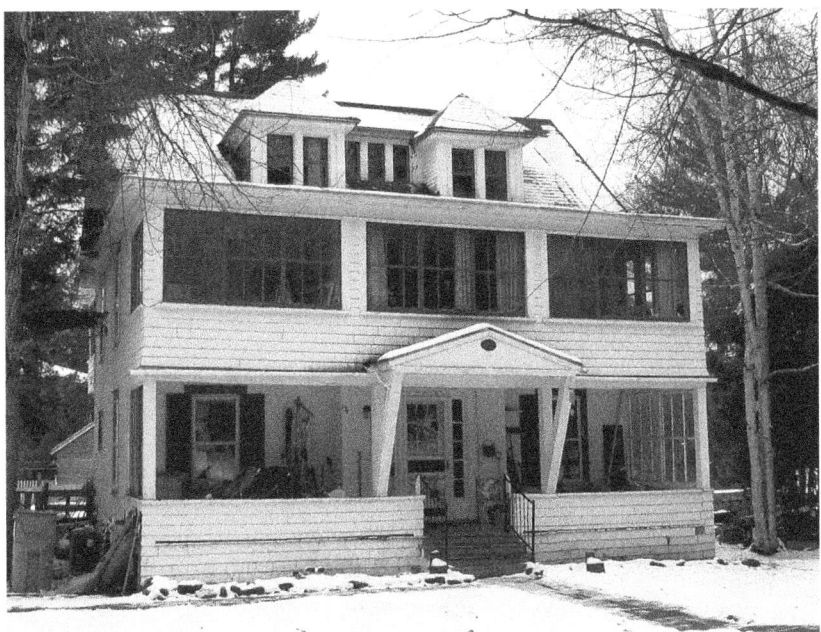

Figure 8.6. Three second-story sleeping porches at the Walker Cottage as it appears today, Saranac Lake, NY. LocalWiKi, https://localwiki.org/hsl/Walker_Cottage.

dollars per week, a sum that rose slightly to eight dollars per week over the years as inflation necessitated (Roberts and Buikstra 2003: 243). By 1894, fewer than ten years after the construction of Little Red, Saranac Lake had 36 buildings dedicated to the cure. Those buildings included an open-air pavilion for recreation, a home for the other resident physician, a library, an administration building, residences for other staff, stables, barns, and infirmary, a laundry, post office, laboratory, workshop, and chapel. During the height of its operation, more than 2,000 patients came to Saranac Lake to cure their tuberculosis (Roberts and Buikstra 2003: 241).

The buildings designed as patient residences were marked by the signature sitting and sleeping porches. A familiar sight at many sanatoria, Saranac Lake included, were groups of people sitting in reclining chairs or rockers on a covered veranda known as a sitting porch. For those bedridden, there was a sleeping porch which was designed to lightly separate patients from the outdoors but also to allow access to abundant sunlight and cold, fresh air (Figure 8.6).

Dr. Lawrason Brown, a leading physician at Saranac Lake, had very specific notions of what made a good cure porch. It should be well ventilated but not drafty, should have movable glass panels on two sides, should face south by southwest in winter and be shaded in summer by deciduous trees. If the patient was not well enough to use the "sitting-out porch," then a "sleeping porch" was recommended. The sleeping porch fulfilled all of the requirements of a sitting-out porch but was connected to the sleeping room by a door wide enough to permit the movement of the bed between the two rooms. It should be located on the second story (Gallos 1985: 8).

Patients rested on cure porches in a specially designed reclining chair/couch known as an Adirondack chair. Dr. Brown, who designed the Adirondack chair, said:

> The chair in which the patient sits out should be the most comfortable in the house. No expense should be spared on it, for here the patient must sit many hours a day. A good chair should elevate the feet from the floor, have a movable back, move easily on casters from place to place, be strongly constructed, and be provided with a good cushion, useful alike for comfort and warmth. . . . A chair of canvas and wood can be had for much [expense] but is not so satisfactory, as it often cramps the shoulders and lungs. . . . Many types of chair can be bought. Personal experience has convinced me that none . . . is more suitable than . . . the "Adirondack Recliner." (Brown 1928: 82)

The Adirondack Recliner was initially manufactured by A. Fortune and Company in Saranac Lake, but before long there were four additional companies that manufactured reclining chairs. The most successful in the end was George L. Starks & Company.

Treatment at TB sanatoria was the preferred method of treatment globally until the 1940s when antibiotics were discovered that could be used to treat the disease. The first antibiotics used were streptomycin and isoniazid (Murray et al. 2015). Chemotherapy rapidly ended the sanatoria movement. Saranac Lake closed the sanatorium in 1954, although the Trudeau Institute at Saranac Lake is still in operation performing biomedical research on lung diseases (Roberts and Buikstra 2003: 247). By 1967, the mortality rate from TB in the United States was reduced to 4.1 per 100,000 (Roberts and Buikstra 2003: 246). It was not just antibiotic treatment, however, but reforms in hygiene, nutrition, and lifestyle. Unfortunately, antibiotic treatments for tuberculosis led to antibiotic resistance, and the current treatment uses a multidrug approach (MDA).

Saranac Lake was but one example of an institutional facility devoted to the care of tuberculous patients. Others, modeled in one way or another after Saranac Lake, were located across America, especially in the western United States. There were also more traditional hospitals in the pavilion plan, large horizontally oriented structures of single, monstrous sanatorium buildings, such as the Peoria Sanatorium in Illinois. Like state hospitals, many of those large buildings have often fallen out of use and into disrepair. They have since lost window glass, plaster, roofs, and been covered with graffiti. Several can be found on YouTube and various paranormal websites as haunted former care facilities. One of the best-known is Waverly Hills in Louisville, Kentucky, which is privately owned and offers tours directed at both those most interested in the actual medical facility and those most interested in the paranormal activity.

* * *

Hospital reform intersected nicely with movements in hygiene, with the acceptance of the germ theory of disease, and with the discovery of specific pathogens. It was not only directed toward physical changes, however, but was extended to an acknowledgment that some conditions required specialized approaches and facilities. Tuberculosis and insanity were two of those conditions which required specialized attention to the diseases, and facilities that placed them in treatment. The hospitals that emerged in the twentieth century were more sterile institutions with a much reduced mortality rate.

IV

The Road to Well-Being, 1850–1900

9

Self-Help Meets Regulation

Patent Medicines, Personal Care, and Professional Regulation

> I am twenty years old and was irregular. I used to be in bed two or three days at a time with a tired, draggy, lonely feeling. A girl at Columbus heard my story and told me about Lydia E. Pinkham's Vegetable Compound. I took one bottle and I noticed the change at once. With this bottle I got a sample of Lydia E. Pinkham's Pills for Constipation. Now during the time that I am indisposed I take these pills. They regulate my bowels and I do not have the headaches any more. I have also used the Sanative Wash and I recommend all these Pinkham products. DAISY JERDON, Shelby, Nebraska.
>
> (Quoted from Lydia Pinkham's Pamphlet *Come into the Kitchen*, No. 151, Summer, 1930: 1)

Mrs. Lydia Estes Pinkham, like many housewives, attended to her family members when they were ill by using medicines made from family recipes or gathered from medical guides, and then made in the home. She drew many of the ingredients from botanical sources, partly stimulated no doubt by the self-help movement called the Thomsonians, after Samuel Thomson. Like many women, she also freely provided her medical cures to people outside of the family. However, in 1873 when a financial depression struck the United States, Lydia Pinkham felt the need to provide financial stability for her family. Mr. Pinkham was largely a failed real estate entrepreneur, and the depression simply made money woes worse.

In the cellar of the Pinkham house in Lynn, Massachusetts, bottles were filled with one of Lydia's favorite vegetable compounds. It was directed at women and women's complaints, and Lydia maintained that only a woman knows about women's ills. She advertised her compound widely, known as *Lydia E. Pinkham's Vegetable Compound,* and her portrait, signed "Yours for Health, Lydia E. Pinkham" adorned the label (Figure 9.1). *Lydia Pinkham's*

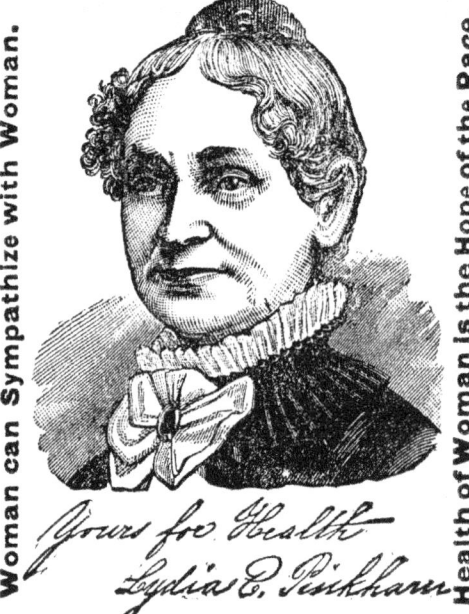

Figure 9.1. Lydia Pinkham's Vegetable Cure advertisement, 1882.

Vegetable Compound bridged the gap between those cures made and consumed within the household and those commercially distributed and widely advertised. It did so because people felt good about Lydia and her compound.

Unlike many other "cures," the Vegetable Compound contained no opium or cocaine. Like many of the other cures, it did contain a robust amount of alcohol, 18 percent (it was later reduced to 15 percent). During Lydia's lifetime, there were several aspects of the business and her compounds that made them appealing to the home consumer. The compounds were home-brewed and the business was run by the family. Lydia wrote most of the advertising herself, and the family recognized that advertising was important. For many years, about half of the profits went back into advertising. Included in the marketing was an invitation to write to Mrs. Pinkham for advice, medical and on other matters. Lydia answered the letters herself on a typewriter. She also wrote a 62-page booklet, *A Guide for Women,* that was translated eventually into five languages.

Patent Medicines: Specialist in a Bottle

What Lydia Pinkham did was to create a proprietary home cure and widely distribute it, and she was only one of hundreds to thousands of manufacturers of such home cures. None were regulated until the Pure Food and Drug Act of 1906, and the ingredients that went into them could largely remain hidden, their effectiveness unknown, and their claims for healing various conditions unproven. Lydia Pinkham provided the ingredients on the bottle, a practice way ahead of its time, and her vegetable compound was largely organic. There was, in fact, support for many of the claims made about ingredients curing specific conditions because she adapted her recipe from King's *American Dispensatory,* a popular medical text at the time.

Lydia Pinkham's Vegetable Compound was immensely successful; at the time of her death in 1883, the compound was bringing in $300,000 per year (Armstrong and Armstrong 1991: 165). Assuming an average inflation rate of 2.39 percent per year (U.S. Dept. of Labor Statistics 2020), that would be $7,666,782 in the currency of 2020. In fact, it was said she was the best-known female face in America. By 1925, sales were up to $3 million in the currency of that time. The company remained run by the family until Lydia's heirs sold it in 1968 to Cooper Laboratories, a pharmaceutical firm. Although Cooper relocated the manufacturing to Puerto Rico in 1972,

Lydia Pinkham's Vegetable Compound is now made in Edison, New Jersey, by Numark Laboratories (Munsey 2003).

Patent medicines were one of the foremost facilitators of healing without seeing a specialist. They were not really patented in the formal way that the Pure Food and Drug Act provided after 1906, but the term was a holdover from the granting of royal patents in Europe for medicine makers (Armstrong and Armstrong 1997: 159; Young 1961). Patent medicines came to America with the British, who in the seventeenth century were accustomed to consuming them from a wide array of available brews. Those of British manufacture dominated the market in America until the revolutionary years; as the American Revolution was gearing up, so was the manufacturing of American patent medicines.

From the outset, the European pharmacopoeia was more focused on mineral and chemical compounds than either those of the Indians or Africans. Non-Europeans were more likely to use botanical compounds, and they did not distinguish between medical practice and pharmaceutical practice. However, European medical traditions did emphasize the link between disease and local environment, and so the knowledge of which plants to use for particular ailments in America came from American Indians. After all, many indigenous plants had been used in America for a considerable time, and they were easy to obtain in fresh form rather than either waiting for weeks or using dried plants. As well, native plants were cheap as compared to the immense cost of imported ingredients.

Indian plant knowledge spanned uses for a wide variety of conditions (Vogel 1970). Astringents to reduce swelling included hemlock, the bark of oak trees, bayberries, and wild geraniums. There were plants to reduce fever (febrifuges) such as the wildflower boneset. Emetic plants that purged the system by inducing vomiting such as hellebore roots had long been used by the Iroquois, as were cathartic laxatives, such as the mayapple. Plants that expelled intestinal parasites, "vermifuges," such as pink root (Indian Pink) were also well known to native populations. Sassafras became widely known as a cure for coughs, bladder pain, and as a blood purifier. Initially used to flavor beer in Pennsylvania, it of course was used to flavor a soft drink as "root beer." Plant-based medicinal compounds became a household necessity in America, and real estate documents from the colonies in the 1700s mention medicinal gardens on estates to be a highly desirable advantage (Gill 1972: 43). Some of those home cures ended up in the patent medicine business.

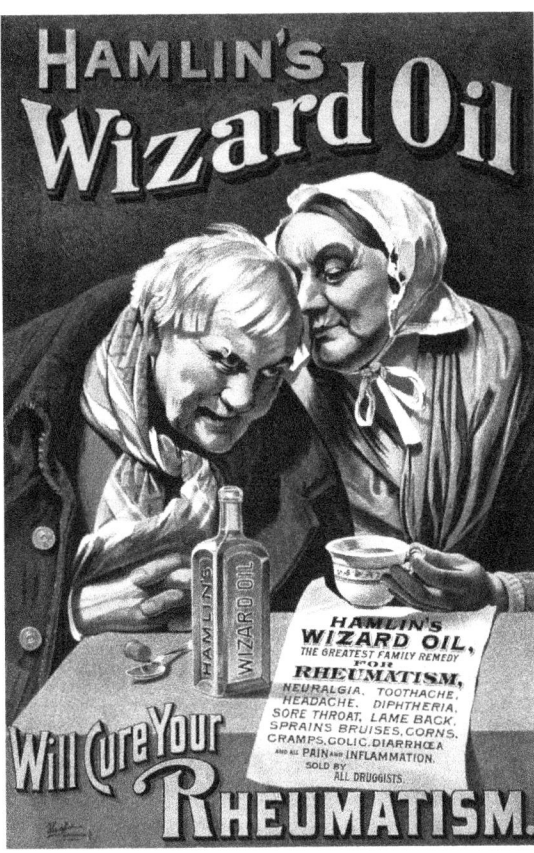

Figure 9.2. Hamlin's Wizard Oil advertisement.

Whether patent medicines were packaged in bottles or tins or pill boxes, they provided homemade cures for many things that ailed a person. Patent medicines combined the preparation of home cures with massive advertising and distribution. Many would contend, in fact, that the advertising was probably more important than the actual ingredients—the ads generally never failed to contain, proudly displayed in large print, the name of the maker. There were Hostetter's Celebrated Stomach Bitters and many other brands of bitters, known for the bitter vegetables and minerals suspended in alcohol. There were Lloyd's Cocaine Tooth Drops, Roger's Cocaine Pile Remedy, Ayer's Cathartic Pills, Paine's Celery Compound, William Radam's Microbe Killer, Hamlin's Wizard Oil, Dr. Sweet's Infallible Liniment, Warner's Safe Cure, Allcock's Porous Plasters, Vegetine the Great Blood Purifier, LeGear's Screw Worm Killer, Dr. William's Pink Pills for Pale People, Carter's Little Liver Pills, and many others (Figure 9.2).

Patent medicine bottles appear in great quantities and numerous contexts, demonstrating the importance of self-treatment in the nineteenth century. It was not that professional medical providers were not involved, but rather it was the context in which the medicines were provided. When medicines were made to order by either physicians or apothecaries, they generally were packaged in embossed bottles with the name of the pharmacy, or in glass bottles with paper labels. Patent medicines were prepackaged in bottles, tins, and pill boxes with the name of the maker on them. They were designed to be taken under the direction of the consumer. Their dosage and periodicity of treatment fell completely in the hands of the individual or household.

The patent medicine bottles found at the Medical College of Georgia (see Chapter 4) dispensary provide an example of the breadth of products (Duncan 1997). Sixty-one embossed bottles were found that had 29 different patent names. Seventeen of those bottles could be linked to specific ailments. The most frequent were medicines to treat consumption, which contained either cherry as a main ingredient (Dr. Wistar's Balsam, Ayer's Cherry Pectoral) or cod liver oil (John C. Baker and Co., Burnett's Cod Liver Oil, Hazard and Caswell Chemists, and Hegeman and Co. Chemists). Upset stomachs were prevalent in the nineteenth century, and medicines to treat that ailment were the next most frequent type of bottle. They include two medicines: Trommer's Extract of Malt Co. and Horlick's Malted Milk. Other intestinal treatments included F. Brown's Essence of Jamaica Ginger and Dr. Henley's California IXL Bitters (Duncan 1997: 60–70).

Other medicines probably had broader application, such as Dr. McMunn's Elixir of Opium, Pond's Extract, and Barnes's Magnolia Water. Dr. McClean's Strengthening Cordial and Blood Purifier was likely used for purification purposes. Interestingly, only one patent medicine treated conditions outside of the body—Holmes's Fragrant Frostilla for the Toilet, used as a skin lotion for chapped hands. As an assemblage, the bottles found in the Medical College of Georgia excavations give a window into the breadth of not only patent medicines, but also of the predominant medical conditions they treated, at least in Augusta.

Apothecary Shops

The distribution of patent medicines was often through apothecaries, businesses specializing in the distribution of medical cures and devices. Apothecaries (the people, not the establishment) generally learned their trade through apprenticeships. There were pharmacy schools; the earliest was the Philadelphia College of Pharmacy established in 1821 (Flannery 2017: 25). There were five others by 1859, all but one located east of the Allegheny mountains. However, apothecary schools were never as popular as medical schools, and most apothecaries did not attend one. Even those that did attended courses generally at night and worked in apothecary shops during the day.

The average apothecary was not as elevated in status as a physician, who had formal university training, yet the two practitioners held much in common. For one, both sets of people compounded medicines. Physicians frequently compounded their own medicines, especially in more rural areas, but they also felt that the trade of apothecary was not one suited for a gentleman. Second, those colonial physicians who had their prescriptions compounded in an apothecary shop often owned the shop and employed an apothecary as a tradesman.

The first documented American apothecary shop was owned by William Davice and was located in Boston in 1646. By 1721, there were 14 apothecary shops in Boston (Gill 1972: 30). Apothecary shops at that time carried an array of goods, as indicated in a *Boston News-Letter* advertisement in March 1712 for Zabdiel Boylston's shop. Boyleston advertised that he had fruit, spice, household sugar, snuff, indigo, eating oil, perfume, painters colors, patent medicines, cupping glasses, nipple shields, urinals, lancets, surgeon's instruments, and "Fresh Druggs and Medicines both Galenical and Chymical, by the last Ship (Capt. Charnock) from London. And in the same Ship had come over a Journey man Apothecary, who for any ones particular occasion can make Dr. Salmon's Medicines, or other preparations in Chymistry" (Gill 1972: 30–31).

Many apothecaries acted as doctors in some contexts as well, and so their shops contained not only tools for preparing and dispensing medicines, but also instruments for tooth extractions and other routine operations. Most apothecary shops therefore contained a few rooms—one for displaying and dispensing medicines, one for compounding medicines, and one for consultation and surgery. Among the things that would be found in the shop are containers of various sizes, a few of which in the eighteenth century were often displayed in a ceramic delftware jar of bright colors. More common were containers of glass, both for storage and dispensing of medicines. The same earthenware gallipots used in household remedies also commonly were used in apothecary shops for storage. Every good apothecary shop kept a fresh supply of leeches, which were dispensed to draw out toxins in the blood, often housed in a nice delftware jar.

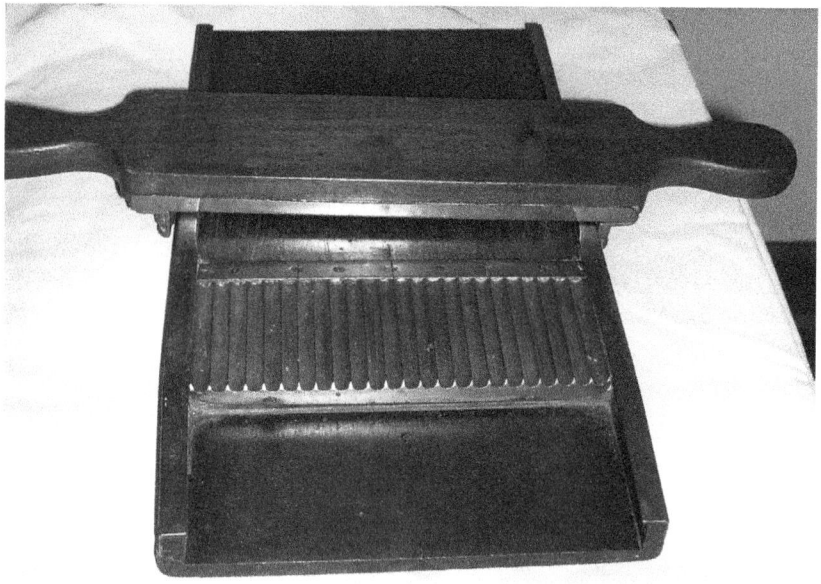

Figure 9.3. Pill roller. Photographed by the author at the Country Doctor Museum, Bailey, NC.

Mortars and pestles of various sizes were used to grind and mix compounds. Most apothecary shops of the eighteenth century contained a still for distilling liquids and oils (see Figure 2.2). Scales were necessary for weighing ingredients and final products. Marble slabs were often used to mix the ingredients for pills as well as for salves and ointments. Pills were among the most labor intensive of medicines to prepare. The ingredients had to be mixed together, and then frequently turned into a paste which would be pressed into pill "logs" and then rolled into uniform sections using a pill roller (Figure 9.3). The pill roller essentially had a grooved surface onto which a grooved upper portion pressed the pill log into uniform sections.

If you were to go into an apothecary in the mid- to late 1800s, you would find a vast array of merchandise for sale. A perfect example of such a shop is the Stabler-Leadbeater shop in Alexandria, Virginia, which opened in 1796 and is still standing and open for visitation as a museum. The shop was opened by Edward Stabler in 1796 in a building that had been built in 1774. Stabler rented the building at first and then purchased it in 1805; he purchased the building next door in 1829. Stabler began his working life as an apprentice to a tanner, but then went to work in the apothecary shop owned by his brother William in Leesburg. He apparently had an earlier shop from 1792 until 1796, but the location of that earlier one is unknown.

The Stabler-Leadbeater shop went through a succession of later owners, first with Edward's son, William, who became an apothecary in 1808, then William's brother-in-law, John Leadbeater, and then down the family line. It was in continuous family operation until 1933. During its days of retail operation, you could find patent medicines at Stabler-Leadbeater, but also cosmetics, medical instruments, insecticides and rat killer, paint, soft drinks, and a host of other things.

The shop had a display area on the first floor (Figure 9.4). However, the upstairs was even more interesting, for that was where the medical library

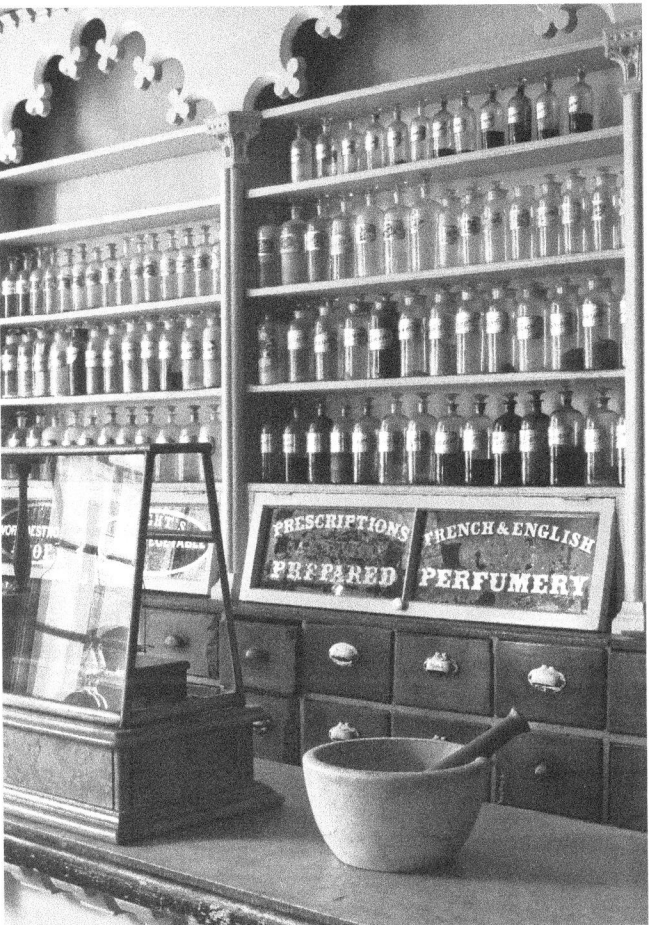

Figure 9.4. Stabler-Leadbeater apothecary display. Used by permission of Stabler-Leadbeater Apothecary Museum.

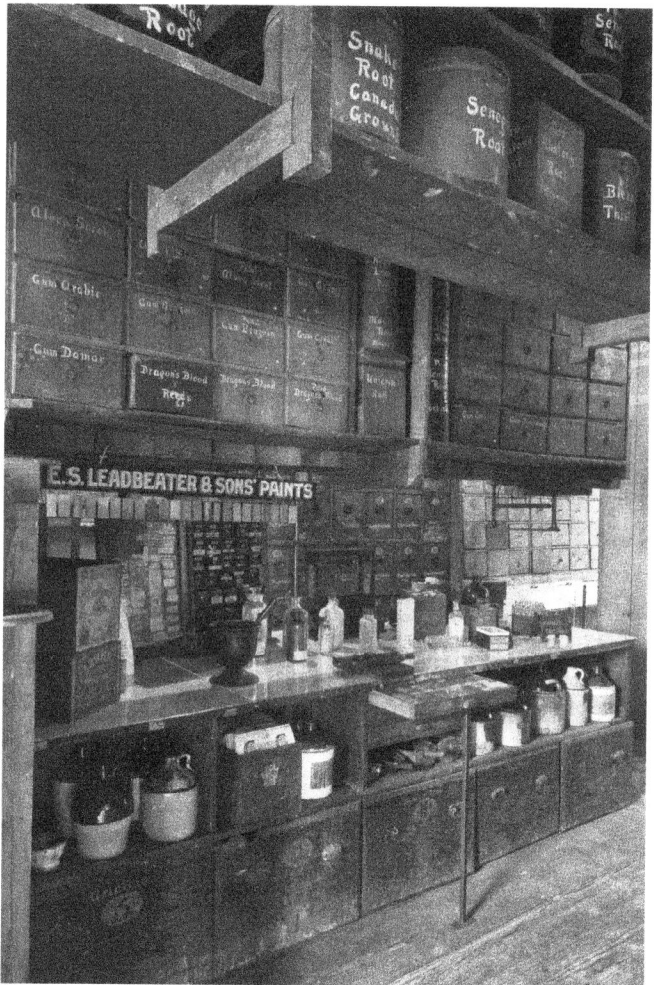

Figure 9.5. Stabler-Leadbeater office and stockroom. Used by permission of Stabler-Leadbeater Apothecary Museum.

was located, a small office, and a very large storage and manufacturing area (Figure 9.5). Numerous bins and containers of herbs lined the shelves, for the shop also was a wholesale distribution point for smaller apothecaries. Anyone familiar with Harry Potter would appreciate the bins and containers labeled dragon's blood, snakeroot, and lovage root. At Stabler-Leadbeater a soft drink beverage was manufactured as were paints. These larger commodities were moved between floors by a mechanical elevator platform located in the floor of the library.

Lawrence Fawcett, a worker in the packing room of the Wholesale Department in 1912, described the shop at that time as a retail shop on the first floor, a second story for wholesale and bottling, and a third floor for storage. A third building to the south was used to make extracts, liniments, and flavors. The largest part of the business was the wholesale part. The largest stock of drugs in the Washington area in 1912 was kept by the Leadbeaters, and they likely distributed them to the nearby six or seven states (Historic Alexandria 2018).

Archaeologists in Alexandria conducted excavations in the cellar of the Stabler-Leadbeater shop between 1982 and 1989 (Historic Alexandria 2018). They investigated two brick-lined shafts, portions of the old earthen floor, and a trash pit that predated the actual building structure. Both brick-lined shafts are thought to be wells, and they contained glass fragments, ceramic sherds, pharmaceutical bottles, ceramic ointment pots, and stoneware jugs. They are all appropriate storage vessels for an apothecary and date to the late nineteenth and early twentieth centuries. In addition to storage vessels, there were glass measuring beakers and metal syringes.

The trash pit contained fragments of plain creamware plates, portions of two delft punch bowls, an earthenware bowl, and part of a teapot. The absence of English pearlware, which was first manufactured in 1775, seems to indicate a date for the other items prior to the 1774 building. Finally, 650 nonhuman animal bones were found in the basement deposits, most from rats which were common inhabitants of Alexandria. There were also, however, bones from rabbit, chicken, beef, sheep, pork, turkey, and fishes, possibly indicating some connection to food processing and distribution.

The archaeological investigation in the Stabler-Leadbeater basement underscores the variety of tasks that were undertaken there. Those tasks ranged from the probable preparation of medicines and their packaging, to the preparation of food, and possibly its consumption. As with many subsurface deposits, they also likely indicate the use of the area for disposal of material items, both organic and inorganic.

Medicine Shows

It would be misleading to discuss the marketing of medical cures and compounds only by considering merchants and storefronts, as some of the most colorful methods of advertising and distribution were medicine shows. Medicine shows ranged in size from a single operator, known as a "pitch doctor" because they delivered a pitch, to large extravagant shows.

Most medicine show performers traveled in wagons, trains, and trucks, and they either slept in their vehicles or camped in tents. They often followed the weather, avoiding colder and snowier climates in the winter when they traveled through the warmer, more southern territories, although some medicine shows did move indoors during the colder times. The places they preferred to perform were parks, vacant lots, opera houses, and fairgrounds.

The medicine show often had a stage with a painted background offering both scenery and advertising. Stages were accompanied by displays of such things as jars of tapeworms and distorted tissue, said to be the possible outcome of ignoring conditions which could be cured by administering the advertised product. The people involved in medicine shows often conducted their presentations with medical charts, anatomical models, and costuming consisting of frocks, coats, top hats, and "Indian" garments. It was common to link their medical compounds to some credible and acknowledged source, such as American Indians, Quakers, or Oriental healers, to name a few. One well-known medicine show was the one that sold Hamlin's Wizard Oil, a liniment made by John A. Hamlin, a magician. Hamlin took Wizard Oil on tour in the 1870s with a host of costumed performers.

Probably the best-known medicine show was the Kickapoo Indian Medicine Company, which acknowledged the contributions of American Indian medical knowledge, but also stigmatized their appearance and behavior. It was run by John Healy and Charles Bigelow out of a tent in front of the train station in Boston from 1881 until 1884, indoors in New York in 1885 and 1886, and finally was based out of Connecticut from 1887 until 1914.

Alongside the stage presentations of the Kickapoo Indian Medicine Company was the sale of their "medical" products which included Kickapoo Cough Syrup, Kickapoo Indian Oil, Kickapoo Worm Expeller, and their best-known product, Kickapoo Indian Sagwa, advertised as a cure for dyspepsia and rheumatism, but having largely a laxative effect. No less recognized a person than Buffalo Bill Cody endorsed the latter product by saying, "An Indian would as soon be without his horse, gun or blanket as without Sagwa" (Armstrong and Armstrong 1991: 178). At the height of its success, the Kickapoo Indian Medicine Company had over 100 different units working in different parts of America, and they had over 4,000 Indians employed as part of the stage presentations (Anderson 2000).

Regulations and Requirements

The tensions between physicians, apothecaries, and midwives, combined with the public distrust of medical professionals and resulting alternative health movements, ensured the inevitable push for regulations and requirements. All the stakeholders had lots to gain by prevailing in their own fields. The reduction of medical school standards, the Jacksonian social movement against elitism, and several competing alternative medical options in the mid-nineteenth century all engendered defensive postures by physicians. Too many people, making too many over-the-counter products, and distributing them outside of standard merchant operations, meant that too many people were getting too much of the pie.

Regulating Patent Medicines

Patent medicines offered people the chance to practice medicine at home, without a specialist, and to seek a self-help cure almost immediately (Young 1961). In the words of James Harvey Young, "Americans have been especially impatient about illness. They have wanted something done—and soon—and have been prone to take things into their own hands, *not* consulting physicians, *before* consulting physicians, *while* consulting physicians. This was true in Lydia Pinkham's day, and the attitude continues" (Young 1977: 111). Self-help, however, reduced the necessity for the service of professional physicians, and physicians fought very hard to regulate non–formally trained practitioners.

It is not surprising that physicians and apothecaries would have some rivalries as well, and they have a deep history. For a long time, there was a distinction made and an emphatic acknowledgment that physicians were university-trained, while apothecaries learned their trade through apprenticeships. Probably the first hint of a formal distinction between physicians and apothecaries appeared in the "Act for Regulating the Fees and Accounts of the Practicers of Physic" in 1736. It made a clear distinction between the fees to be paid to surgeons and apothecaries who served an apprenticeship and those persons "who have studied phistic in any university and taken any degree therein" (see Gill 1972: 24–26, for a full presentation of the Act). The university-trained physician was paid roughly twice as much. In sum, university-trained physicians were generally seen as professionals and apothecaries as members of the trades. This distinction was not universal; at the Pennsylvania Hospital in the mid-eighteenth century, the highest-paid and most prestigious post was that of apothecary (Williams 1976).

In the last quarter of the nineteenth century, physicians, pharmacists and "legitimate" pharmaceutical manufacturers, and journalists began to campaign against the patent medicine trade. Many medical historians point to a series of investigative articles by Samuel Hopkins Adams between 1905 and 1907 that were published in *Collier's Weekly* as an important turning point in patent medicine legislation. Aimed at exposing "quackery," Adams's articles had the title "The Great American Medical Fraud," which fueled a campaign for greater transparency and control of patent medicines.

Attention was also placed on the contents of the elixirs and tonics administered by the nonspecialists—for most patent medicines, the contents were generally not revealed to the consumer. Many contained opium and alcohol, some at extremely high levels. Hostetter's Stomach Bitters, for instance, contained 44.3 percent alcohol, nearly the same as whiskey at 50 percent. Another issue was the simple fact that if people relied on patent medicines, which through their pain-killing contents made them feel better, they did not seek medical intervention for conditions that could be serious.

Prior to regulatory laws, the claims of conditions that could be cured by various patent medicines were often staggering. Even *Lydia E. Pinkham's Vegetable Compound*, with its somewhat restricted claims, offered quite a list of ills cured:

> It will cure entirely the worst form of Female Complaints, all ovarian troubles, Inflammation and Ulceration, Falling and Displacements, and the consequent Spinal Weakness, and is particularly adapted to the Change of Life.
>
> It will dissolve and expel tumors from the uterus in an early stage of development. The tendency to cancerous humors there is checked very speedily by its use.
>
> It removes faintness, flatulency, destroys all craving for stimulants, and relieves weakness of the stomach. It cures Bloating, Headaches, Nervous Prostration, General Debility, Sleeplessness, Depression and Indigestion.
>
> That feeling of bearing down, causing pain, weight and backache, is always permanently cured by its use. It will at all times and under all circumstances act in harmony with the laws that govern the females system. For the cure of Kidney Complaints of either sex this Compound is unsurpassed. (*Lydia Pinkham's Vegetable Compound* advertisement, 1882; see Figure 8.1)

The Pure Food and Drug Act of 1906 represented the first attempt to regulate patent medicines by requiring manufacturers to list the ingredients on the label. That single requirement resulted in the removal of large numbers of claims. Kickapoo Indian Oil, for instance, went from pre-1906 "A safe, sure and speedy relief for all nervous and inflammatory diseases. A quick cure for all kinds of pain; for toothache, headache, earache, sore throat, chilblains, burns, freezes, cuts, sprains, bruises, neuralgia and rheumatic pains, colic, cholera morbus, diarrhoea, dysentery, croup, and all sudden or acute pains, external or internal" to post-1906 "the relief of aches and pains" after the Act was passed (Young 1961).

In 1938, the Food, Drug, and Cosmetic Act further stipulated that drugs had to be proven safe before they were released on the market. Labels had to include directions for proper use and information misuse. The revision of the Food, Drug, and Cosmetic Act in 1962 took further actions to protect the consumer by extending regulation beyond safety to effectiveness; claims that a product produced a specific result had to be demonstrated.

Midwives, Medicines, and Malpractice

Despite the preponderance of midwives and a general feeling that birth was a woman's affair, after about 1760 American male doctors began to share delivery responsibilities (Berman 1990). One of the first and most famous male obstetricians was William Shippen who began practice in 1763. Shippen learned the techniques of obstetrical medicine in Europe at the medical school in Edinburgh, and he trained many others in those techniques. Elite women in Philadelphia, where Shippen was located, as well as women in other colonial urban centers, began increasingly to choose physicians for their obstetrical needs and a class structure in birthing emerged (Leavitt 1986: 36–40).

Midwives and physicians practiced in parallel between roughly 1760 and 1950, but there was often tension between the two types of specialists. Trained physicians stressed their medical knowledge and specialized tool kit—the most recognized tools were the obstetrical forceps. Forceps had been used in Europe since the 1730s, and they facilitated grasping the child high in the birth canal for easing out or repositioning the head. Midwives saw the practice as brutal, emphasizing their gentle hands as compared to the iron forceps. They further emphasized that having males in the birthing room compromised women's privacy. In turn, physicians cast suspicions that midwives were colluding with women to provide illegal abortions.

By the nineteenth century, attention to the moral and legal concerns about abortion circulated throughout the medical community. In response, Britain and Ireland passed laws against aborting a quickened fetus. In 1821, Connecticut became the first state in the United States to outlaw aborting quickened fetuses (Wilkie 2003: 149). Quickening, however, was still a difficult measure of pregnancy because it usually could only be applied in the second trimester; the invention of the stethoscope in 1818 by Théophile-René-Hyacinthe Laënnec changed all of that. Through the new device, physicians could detect a fetal heartbeat, and thus confirm pregnancy much earlier than the second trimester (Riddle 1997). That said, the stethoscope did not routinely enter American medical practice until after 1860.

Birth control also became a topic of discussion in the second half of the nineteenth century, as did family planning and abortion. It had long been suspected, and fairly well demonstrated, that many plants could terminate a pregnancy. Although most of the plants used as emmenagogues were initially grown by family and friends in gardens and fields, by the end of the eighteenth century increasing population density restricted access of urban women to gardens.

Domestic preparation of emmenagogic compounds gave way to commercial ones, often known as "female pills" or "female tonics." Entire medical chests could be purchased which contained numerous assortments of herbs, patent medicines, and prepared drugs. Apothecaries carried a number of plants and other compounds that they dispensed in a number of forms. By about 1850, new methods of contraception concentrated on methods linked to intercourse, such as withdrawal, abstinence, barrier methods (sponges, cervical caps, condoms), douches, and sponges.

Following on earlier laws regulating birth control and abortions, the passage of the 1873 Comstock Act was intended to prevent doctors from providing advice on birth control. Without the advice of doctors, women turned increasingly to patent medicines that provided assistance with "female problems," including birth control and pregnancy. After about 1875, more patent medicines for "ladies complaints" were incorporated into the midwife tool kit, although they did not necessarily replace earlier homemade cures.

Among the most common of those female-directed patent medicines was *Lydia Pinkham's Vegetable Compound, Dr. Worden's Female Pills for all Female Diseases,* and *Brown's Vegetable Cure for Female Weakness.* Folk remedies also provided women with help restoring menses. Midwives were likely the most numerous healers who provided home remedies, and they increasingly became the subject of charges by physicians (especially through the American Medical Association) that they were aiding in abortions.

Midwives, however, were not the only health practitioners aiding in birth control or abortions. As pointed out in several earlier discussions, there is both historical and archaeological evidence of the involvement of male physicians performing gynecological tasks and treatments.

* * *

Lucrecia Perryman provides an interesting case study of a midwife in the late nineteenth and early twentieth centuries. She lived in Mobile, Alabama, and was active as a nurse and midwife from at least 1892 through her retirement in about 1910 or 1911 (all information regarding the Perryman site comes from Wilkie 2003). The site of the Perryman house was on the property of Crawford Park in Mobile, Alabama. It was excavated in 1994 during landscaping and expansion of the park. Construction and landscape grading unfortunately removed some of the midden materials, and thus some of the archaeological record was lost.

There were, however, two subsurface features that provided a glimpse into the Perrymans' lives. The first was a trash pit that likely dates to around 1885; it was filled largely with glass and ceramic fragments. The second was a well that seems to have been filled in during one large episode around 1909 or 1910. The well deposit was 130 cm (51.2 inches; 4.27 feet) deep and contained a large number of glass medicine bottles, jars, and vials representing the period from about 1890 through 1910, the period of Lucrecia's midwifery.

The trash pit and well contain material culture that transcends a period of male obstetricians and midwives practicing in parallel, a period of suspicions about the possible illegal activities of midwives. The materials in the well date to Lucrecia's midwife practice, and because it was a trash depository, one could assume that if she were trying to hide something, it would be a likely repository. A minimum of 122 glass medical containers were recovered from the well, 83 of which were embossed with brand names.

None of these containers was identifiable as those containing formulas for "female problems." Thirty-five local pharmacy bottles from seven different pharmacies were recovered. Twenty-seven of those were from one pharmacy, Antwerp's Pharmacy. Also found were 25 large stoneware whiskey jugs and 25 stoneware gin bottles. At least 51 liquor bottles and flasks were also found. Ten bottles were extract bottles that contained various extracts of peppermint, lemon, ginger, and vanilla. There were a dozen glass scrapers, a vaginal pipe for a syringe kit, and a number of Vaseline jars.

Wilkie (2003) interprets the material evidence to indicate that Lucrecia Perryman was making her own medicines. She was buying some of the ingredients and then combining them to form her own household remedies, which she administered to her patients out of her house. The pharmacy bottles, the extracts, the whiskey, and a number of faunal remains, all are consistent with their use as ingredients for home cures. The pharmacy bottles were likely then reused to contain the homemade "tonics." The flasks and liquor bottles likely represent alcohol for home enjoyment. There were also two containers that indicate the care of children's nutrition, *Horlick's Malted Milk* and *Mellin's Infant's Food*. No nursing bottles were found.

In sum, Lucrecia was likely making a number of medicines by combining ingredients, both for child nutrition and for medical complaints of children and mothers. The ingredients of some may have been used for birth control or abortion, but it is unclear if that is the case. No patent medicines that might aid in birth control or to stimulate abortion were found. One could infer from the materials found that Lucrecia, like many midwives, offered care in health and well-being that spanned women's reproductive health in a number of ways and included the early care of children.

* * *

Patent medicines represented the ultimate push for self-help in the form of over-the-counter medications. They were not regulated in terms of content, or the claims made about the conditions for which they provided remedies. The unregulated manufacture of patent medicines, as well as the unsubstantiated claims made about their effects, necessitated oversight. Unlike dietary restrictions, hygiene, or physical exercise, patent medicines were centered on the ingestion of substances that at times were unhealthy, if not dangerous.

Regulations placed through the chain of food and drug acts were part of the larger struggle between formally trained specialists and other health practitioners. In the case of patent medicines, the oversight was justified because patent medicines differed from traditional medicines through their marketing and availability. Regulation was probably inevitable.

There was more to the resistance against patent medicines, though, and to non–formally trained medical specialists, and that was largely about competition and legitimization. Physicians, formally trained and licensed to practice, often competed with those whose expertise was not formally recognized or filtered through trade associations. The Pure Food and Drug Act, while absolutely necessary, facilitated the legitimacy of formally trained physicians and the rise of institutional health care.

10

Making Oneself Better

Vitamins, Diet, Exercise, and Other Fads

> One individual, who had just been confined, but was a little feverish, consented not only to drink cold water, but be sponged with it. Not, indeed, when the "fever was off," as the saying is, but during the time of the highest excitement. Cold water, in this instance, acted like a charm. Not a week elapsed, if I recollect rightly, before she was able to bathe in cold water in the usual manner, and with entire safety. Since that time she does not hesitate to bathe regularly, down to the day of her confinement, and to resume it as soon as all is over.
>
> (Alcott 1845: 21)

Sylvester Graham may have been an early voice for dietary confinement, but he was certainly joined by many others. Several people built upon his vegetarianism, but one of the most notable was Dr. William Alcott. Whether it be the botanics, or the homeopaths, or the Thomsonians, they all generally chartered paths away from formally trained physicians and toward self-help, albeit sometimes guided through spas and sanatoria. The popular movements they sponsored urged people interested in their health to think about what you eat, how you eat it, and how to practice a healthy physical life. In a sense, they gave people back their lives, because only you can practice your diet and lifestyle, and following the Civil War, Americans were ready to have more control in their own lives.

Making Oneself Better through Food

Neither strictly vegetarian nor vegan diets by themselves became prominent movements in America until the twentieth century, but vegetarianism did play a role in many popular health-reform movements. The Seventh-day Adventists were one of those groups that adopted a meat-free diet in 1863, largely through the Graham dietary plan. From Battle Creek, Michigan, they published the periodical *Advent Review and Sabbath Herald,* and built the foundations of the Seventh-day Adventist Church.

It wasn't just what you ate for dietary reformists, but how much, how often, and just plain how. Seventh-day Adventists took two meals per day, an early 7 a.m. breakfast and 1 p.m. dinner. They followed Graham's insistence on unrefined grains, fruits, and vegetables. There was no alcohol and no gluttony. It was Horace Fletcher, however, who went beyond the how-much and how-often to just plain *how.* Fletcher preached the power of mastication in making food as nutritious as possible. Saliva, Fletcher reasoned, is needed to mix the food and release the nutrients. Chewing should occur until the food is liquified, all the flavor gone, and held in the mouth for at least 30 seconds after liquification, a process John Harvey Kellogg called "Fletcherizing."

While everyone recognized that the best way to obtain the proper nutrients was to eat the foods containing them, there were still those who advocated "supplements" just in case. Vitamin supplements were, however, largely a post–nineteenth century phenomenon. Vitamins (and minerals), as we know them, did not really emerge as a market item until the 1940s, after Szent-Györgyi won a Nobel prize for his study of vitamin C in 1934, and about the same time as Edward Doiry won another Nobel prize for isolating vitamin K.

There had been earlier contributions—Casimir Funk found in 1911 that the mystery substance behind beriberi was thiamine, vitamin B1. Funk went beyond the connection between thiamine and beriberi to postulate that several other deficiency diseases (scurvy, rickets, and pellagra) were caused by similar vitamin deficiencies, although supportive proof came much later (Armstrong and Armstrong 1991: 237). He also coined a term for the substances, "vitamine"—*vita* for life and *amine* for nitrogen-containing substances. Despite the fact that vitamins aren't amines, the term stuck for quite awhile until finally it was shortened to vitamin.

The scientific discovery of vitamins sketched out above, however, leaves one with a completely false picture. Native Americans knew well ahead of the European entry into America that the condition where one bleeds internally, or develops lesions of the gums, or when one's joints swell could be prevented by consuming spruce. Jacques Cartier learned of the use of spruce to cure scurvy from Indians near Montreal in 1536 (Biggar 1924: 204–215). They showed him how to grind the bark and leaves and boil them in water to form a drink which almost immediately allowed his men to recover, but not before 25 had died of the mysterious condition.

Making Oneself Better through Water

> In the beginning the colonists visited mineral springs for their health, rich and poor alike, according to their means. However, as certain springs acquired tone, the well-to-do traveled to places that were exclusive and where they could meet people of their own kind. Not only did the waters of such resorts have therapeutic value, but the rest and recreation and change of scene were stimulating and beneficial. The exclusive mineral springs became centers of society seeking change, romance, adventure, health, and relief from boredom, according to one's age. Of course, the fashionable maladies were the gout, the vapors, and phthisis. (Weiss and Kemble 1962: 21)

People came to mineral water spas for two reasons: to cure health problems and as a preventive measure. Before the Civil War, the clientele was largely comprised of those needing curing, but after the war the spas became fashionable gathering spots for society's elite.

The use of water as a curative agent has a long history in many cultural traditions. Galen, the Roman physician, wrote of the power of cold water for curing fevers. Ice water and wet linens were used in China for a variety of afflictions. In the middle of nineteenth-century America, therapeutic water cures were the rage. There were two kinds of water therapy in the nineteenth century. The first, known popularly as hydrotherapy, focused on treating illness with ordinary water, through consumption and bathing. The second, often referred to as "taking the waters," involved consumption of and bathing in mineral waters (Green 1986: 140).

Hydropathy was introduced in the 1850s and it involved the consumption of copious amounts of water, often said to be five to six gallons or 20 to 30 glasses per day, and it offered an alternative to alcohol-laced pharmaceuticals. John Harvey Kellogg championed water (not mineral water) as a curative agent in his book *The Uses of Water in Health and Disease* (1876). The consumption of water internally was accompanied by cold water wraps, baths, and dunks (Figure 10.1).

Hydropathy was not limited to cold water, however, and steam rooms, Turkish baths, and other warm water cures were also popular. Water cure treatments were published in the immensely popular tabloid, *The Water-Cure Journal*. For those who could afford it, visits to an establishment specializing in water cures, colloquially known simply as "the Cures," were the height of fashion. The first Cures were located in New York in the 1840s

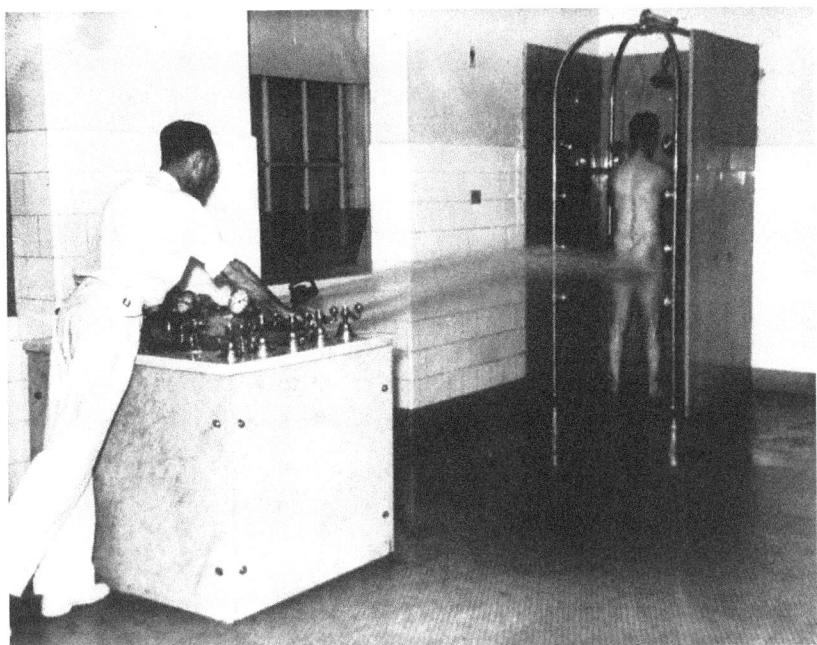

Figure 10.1. Hydropathy treatment: A male patient stands in a shower stall while a physical therapist gives him a heavy spray of water aimed at his back. National Library of Medicine Unique ID: 101447290 (see catalog record); NLM Image ID: A020852.

and were owned by Russell Trall and Joel Shew (Armstrong and Armstrong 1991: 82).

The year 1851 saw the opening of the first hydropathic medical school, Thomas and Mary Gove Nichols's American Hydropathic Institute, which was followed in 1853 by the establishment of Russell Trall's New York Hygeio-Therapeutic College. By 1853, *The Water-Cure Journal* listed 41 Cures, largely located in the state of New York, but Cures emerged later in Pennsylvania, Massachusetts, and New Jersey. Many listed their staff physicians in the advertisements, of which there were no shortage; the time from entrance to a hydropathy college to graduation was a mere three months (Armstrong and Armstrong 1991: 83).

The hydropathy movement was short-lived, and by 1870, it was giving way to mineral water cures; by 1900, most hydropathy Cures had closed. Several of those that remained reformed themselves into sanatoriums focused more on recuperation than on strict dietary regimens and exercise. The waning of hydropathy, however, was not the end of water as a curative agent, and in the last half of the nineteenth century mineral water was heralded for its restorative powers. Like the use of nonmineral water emphasized by hydrologists, mineral water cures had a lengthy history. Both the Greeks and Romans enjoyed warm mineral baths, as did Native Americans (Weiss and Kemble 1962: 9–19).

* * *

The late 1860s saw a change in how Americans chose to take care of their health. The sanitary commissions that were established during the Civil War, the microbial analysis of the causes of disease, and increased home sanitation were all connected to a decline in hydropathic water cures and increased attention to mineral water consumption and bathing. Across America, mineral water was bottled or consumed on site, and mineral water resorts sprang up across America after 1865. Unlike hydropathic Cures which catered primarily to the sick, mineral springs tended to cater to those of financial means, often urban dwellers, who were just worn out and stressed. By the end of the nineteenth century, "spas," as mineral spring resorts came to be known, provided numerous forms of entertainment and many necessary comforts.

Saratoga Springs in New York was one of the popular mineral spring resorts, as was Georgia's Madison Springs, the latter famous for its Southern cooking. The popular spas were no small operations, "In 1850 the United States Hotel at Saratoga had 1,100 persons to feed daily. This number consisted of 700 guests, 100 children, and 300 servants, and each day, in addition to many other articles of food, they consumed 500 pounds of beef, 500 pounds of mutton, 500 chickens, 150 ducks and turkeys, 2,500 eggs, 600 pounds of butter, 1,500 rolls for breakfast, and 4 barrels of flour" (Weiss and Kemble 1962: 25). By 1870, the local population in Saratoga was 8,000, "and a transient summer population in one day as high as 12,000" (Weiss and Kemble 1962: 25). Saratoga offered, in addition to the springs, horse racing and gambling.

Consuming or soaking in mineral water was frequently touted not just as a cure for "nervous exhaustion," or "Neurasthenia Americana," but as a benefit for numerous other conditions. Nervous exhaustion, or American nervousness, was an idea put forth by a number of different health reformers, but was codified by the New York neurologist George M. Beard in his book *American Nervousness* (1881). Beard attributed nervous exhaustion to the socioeconomic transformation that placed more people in urban environments and whose occupations were increasingly as "brain workers" rather than rural physical laborers. He was very clear (mistakenly, of course) that this was a condition of men who had greater cranial capacity and whose intellectual pursuits went beyond the trivial matters that occupied the thoughts of women.

The popular spas certainly did not share the meatless or moderate diet advocated by so many of the popular health movements of the mid- to late 1800s, nor did they eschew the consumption of alcohol or tobacco. Accommodations to treat neurasthenia, after all, had to be luxurious given that the condition affected largely affluent professionals. There were far more spas located in the West, many accessible by railroad, and in 1877 a guide to American hot springs was published by D. Appleton and Company, a publisher of railroad guides (Green 1986: 149). It was followed in 1894 by *Western Resorts for Health and Pleasure Reached via Union Pacific System*.

Archaeological investigations at the Hot Wells Hotel in San Antonio, Texas, offer some glimpses into the material culture associated with a mineral springs resort (Fox and Highley 1985). The excavations were conducted in 1984 by the Center for Archaeological Research at University of Texas–San Antonio. The hotel, built in 1901, had nearly a quarter century of attendance before it burned down in 1925. The large brick building used as a bathhouse for the sulphur springs remained standing at the time of investigation, although it was uninhabitable.

The history of the Hot Wells property begins in 1892 with the discovery of an artesian well containing sulfur water on the property owned by the Southwestern Insane Asylum located a few miles south of San Antonio. Recognizing the medicinal and recreational potential of the well, several entrepreneurs established facilities under a variety of names: Natural Hot Sulphur Wells, Hot Wells Hotel and Bath House, Hotel Hot Sulfur Wells, Hot Wells Park, and others (Fox and Highley 1985: 4). In an early iteration of its business offerings, the property was known as Southwestern Park, and advertising claimed the water, with numerous minerals and a temperature of 104 degrees Fahrenheit, had healing powers for rheumatism, kidney, liver, and skin diseases, in addition to blood poisoning and other diseases.

Following a fire that destroyed most of the first building on the property, the Texas Hot Sulphur Sanitarium Company constructed a natatorium between 1900 and 1901, with three swimming pools (for men, women, and families) and a hotel. In 1902, the hotel was described as a three-story brick structure with a frontage of 200 feet, a tiled, gabled roof, three wings with courtyards in between, and a total of 80 rooms. The rooms had steam heat, electric and gas lights, telephones to the main office, and luxurious furnishings. An addition in 1907 added an extension to the hotel with 90 rooms.

The bathhouse had 45 private bathrooms with tile floors, partitions of marble, and solid porcelain tubs. One could take steam, Turkish, Russian, Roman, needle, and shower baths in separate facilities for men and women. There were masseurs available. Gambling was popular at the hotel, and the gambling rooms and bar were located on the first floor of the bathhouse. Among the guests over the years were Rudolph Valentino, Sarah Bernhardt, Will Rogers, Teddy Roosevelt, J. P. Morgan, and Douglas Fairbanks. Unfortunately, the combined impacts of World War I, Prohibition, and the Depression began to affect the hotel's popularity after 1915. It was sold to the Christian Scientists in 1923 and converted into a school shortly before it burned.

In 1984, archaeologists were able to locate the 1901 hotel building and reconstruct the plan of the hotel and bathhouse, which matched photographs taken of the hotel. The footings for the building extended to a considerable depth, understandable given the size of the building. Artifacts recovered include fine china and glassware used in the hotel, some with the hotel name on it. Interestingly, the ceramics are a mixture of porcelain, earthenware, stoneware, and crocks or churns. Ironstone earthenware was commonly used in hotels and restaurants and a number of different types and patterns were found at Hot Wells Hotel.

The most frequent type of glass found was from clear screw-top beverage and food containers. There were also many brown glass alcoholic beverage and medicine bottles recovered. Much of the glass was melted, presumably from one of the fires on the property. The metal hardware found was ornate, attesting to the many descriptions of the hotel's splendor.

For those who could not afford to go to a spa, the increased attention to bathing after 1850 meant that a spa experience could be had at home in a tub. Home consumption of mineral waters was made possible through advances in bottling technology. One of the most famous bottled spring waters was Excelsior spring water, bottled and sold by A. R. Lawrence and Company in Saratoga Springs.

Making Oneself Better through Electricity

> Electricity is the greatest power on earth. It puts life and force into whatever it touches; gives relief to rheumatism, backache, kidney, liver and bladder troubles, early decay, night losses, lack of nerve and vigor, nervous debility, constipation, dyspepsia, undevelopment and

lost vitality, and all female complications. (U.S. Department of Propaganda for Reform 1915: 1202)

Just about as miraculous, and as eye-catching as fire, is electricity, as portrayed in the Department of Propaganda for Reform's statement, and it did not escape the attention of the self-help, antiphysician movement of the nineteenth century. The idea wasn't new. In the 1770s, Franz Anton Mesmer thought the cause of all disease was an imbalance of invisible electrical fluid (Armstrong and Armstrong 1991: 186). W. R. Wells (1869) later built upon Mesmer's idea and pronounced that all disease is caused by a loss of electrical balance in the diseased part of the body. One simply had to apply electricity to the parts of the body diagnosed as out of balance, and one could restore health, he said.

By the late nineteenth century, electrically assisted medicine and well-being was made possible by a number of contraptions which either instilled into a person good electricity or removed bad electricity. There were electric baths, handheld electrical devices such as combs and brushes, electric cages, electric helmets, and a range of electric belts. Especially attractive were electric belts, often called Galvanic Belts, as they could be worn unseen and could seemingly fix almost anything.

The proponents of electrical therapy saw the human body as one large compound electromagnet from which electricity was constantly escaping. It escaped most from the extremities, especially the feet, because of the circuit they made with the earth. Sleep was time when one had to be particularly careful and one could interrupt that circuit with the earth while sleeping by placing Hall's Glass castors for Insulating Bedsteads under the feet of the bed (Green 1986: 173). The electrical therapy movement was something that involved many devoted people. It was extremely widespread and a number of book-length treatises such as *The Electric Physician* (Britten 1875) and *A Practical Treatise on the Medical and Surgical Uses of Electricity* (Beard and Rockwell 1871) were published to help the electrically devoted patient.

Making Oneself Better through Exercise

Fitness was another part of the health movement in the second half of the nineteenth century. Like many other movements, the fitness movement emphasized avoiding physicians and taking charge of one's health through preventive habits. It also had roots in major changes in American family life as more and more people left rural environments, and the physical labor associated with living off the land, for urban jobs that required less physical labor. Gymnasiums became immensely popular, as did competitive sports. Physical culture became a raging popular movement. Fitness appealed to people because they could do it without necessarily working with a specialist, and like diet it had a preventive quality to it—it emphasized helping to keep it from happening rather than fixing it once it happens.

"The Athletic Revival," as *Harper's Weekly* called it in 1860, embraced the involvement of women and children. William Alcott advocated exercise in playgrounds as a developmental enhancement for the growing youth. Catherine Beecher, in addition to her advice for a healthy home in *American Woman's Home,* penned *Physiology and Calisthenics* (Beecher 1856), which had a substantial emphasis on the biology of the human body.

One of the most vocal proponents of integrating women, children, and the elderly into exercise programs was Dioclesian Lewis, a physical education instructor. Lewis was an early supporter of women's rights, health reform, temperance, and homeopathy. The inclusion of women into exercise programs also undermined the somewhat socially reinforced wearing of the corset. Lewis advocated the wearing of loose clothing when doing calisthenics, and began the reformation of a long-standing practice of wearing corsets. Tight-fitting and confining, corsets had seen many critics of "waists," as they were often called.

While corsets were embraced as the height of fashion until the Roaring Twenties, they physically deformed women's bodies, especially their rib cages, lungs, and spines. Ludovic O'Followell, a French doctor, published books in 1905 and 1908 on the detrimental physical effects of corset wearing. O'Followell's second book in 1908 was novel because it included numerous illustrations of the physical damage caused by corsets, including X-rays (Figure 10.2), a technology which was relatively new (O'Followell 1908). It had been only a little more than a decade before, in 1895, that the X-ray had been discovered by Wilhelm Conrad Röentgen. He was awarded the very first Nobel Prize in Physics for his discovery.

Fitness fanatics of the current time are all about gear; Americans love gear when it comes to fitness and sports. It was no different in the late nineteenth and early twentieth centuries. Gear was accompanied by instructive manuals such as *A Manual of Free Gymnastic and Dumb-Bell Exercises for the School-Room and Parlor* (Stuart 1864) and *New Gymnastics for Men, Women, and Children* (Lewis 1862). Popular pieces of gymnastic equipment included dumbbells, some made of wood, and Indian clubs. Rowing was an

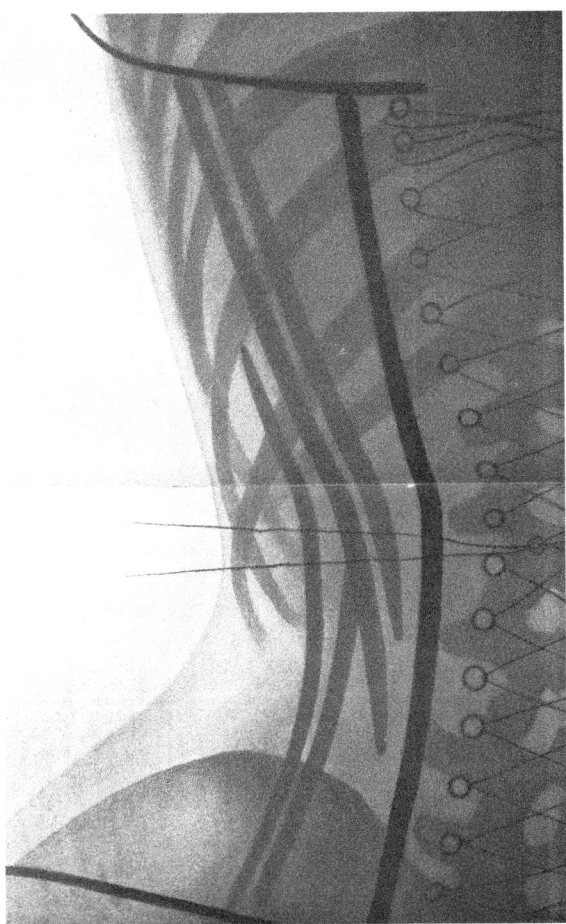

Figure 10.2. Deformed ribs due to corset wearing. From O'Followell 1908, Plate 2.

extremely popular activity in the mid- to late 1800s, and various kinds of parlor rowing machines were situated in homes. Dr. Barnett's Parlor Gymnasium even allowed people to exercise at their desks.

Another of the heroic figures of the exercise movement was Bernarr Macfadden, born in 1868 in Missouri. In his teenage years Bernarr became disillusioned with both drugs and doctors, and, in seeking a way to deal with his weak physical state, found exercise. By eighteen years of age he was teaching gymnastics and preventive health methods that combined fasting, semivegetarianism, fresh air, and long walks (Armstrong and Armstrong 1991: 204).

In 1898, he began publishing a journal version of his preventive advice, *Physical Culture*. As the readership of his magazine grew, so did his followers, and Macfadden became a guru of exercise and health. He opened several restaurants, had a radio fitness program, and wrote several books. His dietary advice generally followed that of Sylvester Graham, although he did include some meat, preferably beef, and he was a strong supporter of the importance of eating dairy products. He stressed that one should not eat unless one is hungry.

Macfadden's *Physical Culture* had reached 500,000 readers by 1918, and by the 1930s he was a New York millionaire, a status that unfortunately was not meant to last. A number of bad political moves led to his financial demise, although he lived to the ripe old age of 88. He undoubtedly influenced a huge number of people; the most well-known of his followers was Charles Atlas.

Making Oneself Better through Guided Practice

Health resorts probably had some roots in the resorts frequented by those seeking to escape malaria during the summer season. They catered mostly to those who could afford the lavish lifestyle and had the time to devote to substantial periods of self-care. In pursuit of health and well-being, the clients of health resorts indulged in focused management of various types of health "problems."

In 1866, the Seventh-day Adventist founder, Ellen G. White, opened an Adventist health resort called the Western Health Reform Institute on eight acres of land near Battle Creek. After a decade of marginal growth, John Harvey Kellogg was hired as the chief physician in 1876. Kellogg had grown up as a Seventh-day Adventist and attained a medical degree. He was an energetic visionary, and despite his young age of 24, he moved quickly to transform the institution, once staffed with Adventist volunteers, into a combination of hospital, spa, lecture hall, and hotel and dining facility. In 1877, a year after he assumed the post, he changed the name to the Battle Creek Sanitarium; it came to be widely known as "the San."

To say John Harvey Kellogg was a dedicated health advocate is to say life is healthier than death. Kellogg was emphatic about his practices, at times a showman, and not gentle in his assertions. Nearly every popular approach to health was in some way incorporated into Kellogg's prescribed treatments at the San. Both hydropathy and electrical stimulation were widely administered.

Exercise was fundamental in Kellogg's health care plan, but only as long as it didn't involve sex. There was neither meat, nor stimulants, nor alcohol. He was known for displaying bodily parasites under the microscope and was devoted to the health of the colon. There were plenty of healthful vegetables and fruits, grains, and John Harvey Kellogg's signature breakfast, corn flakes. So the story goes, an elderly patient at the San complained about the hardness of a biscuit, and seeking a softer breakfast food, Kellogg created the first precooked, flaked cereal in 1894 (Armstrong and Armstrong 1991: 107).

By the early 1890s, the San had been transformed into an elegant health resort (Kellogg 1908). A visit to the San included using the immense gymnastic and spa facilities, and clients were attended to by a host of professional nurses who saw after their treatments. Meals were taken in a fancy dining room with plants and abundant sunlight. The diners ate while a chamber orchestra played, and dinner was usually punctuated by words from the great man himself. All manner of socials occurred on the front lawn, many of which were accompanied by a brass band that played the energetic theme song of the San, "The Battle Creek Sanitarium March."

John Harvey Kellogg's adventures at the San are satirized in a popular novel, *The Road to Wellville,* by T. Coraghessan Boyle (1994) and were later made into a movie with no less a prodigious actor than Anthony Hopkins playing Kellogg. There is a great scene of Matthew Broderick wearing a galvanic belt in *The Road to Wellville.* Both the book and the film illustrate that the San was one of the most well-known and eccentric of the centers for elite health and well-being.

Kellogg's transformation of the San into the premier boarding salon for the wealthy continued to take place when Ellen G. White lived abroad in Australia and New Zealand between 1891 and 1900. When she returned, she was dismayed to find her Seventh-day Adventist health center was a secular business. After a period of contention, during which she predicted the San would be visited by a sword of fire, it burned down in 1902. Kellogg rebuilt it as a five-story building in Italian Renaissance style, with a solarium, roof garden, marble floors, and a glass-domed palm garden (Figure 10.3). Kellogg and Sister White at that point were at complete odds, and although Sister White had Kellogg removed from the church in 1907, he maintained control of the San until his death in 1943.

It might seem as if John Harvey Kellogg was a shameless promotional genius, but he was also a dedicated and insightful physician, albeit more than a little forceful in his opinions. Kellogg was acclaimed for his surgery, and such notable surgeons as William and Charles Mayo came to view his surgical techniques. He reportedly made the connection between smoking tobacco and lung cancer decades before it was demonstrated. Ahead of his

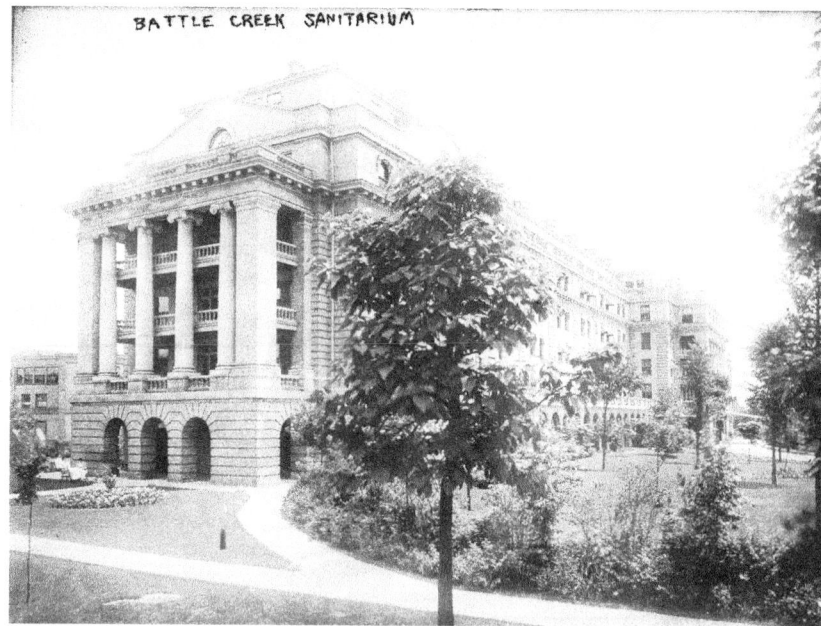

Figure 10.3. Exterior view of the Battle Creek Sanitarium between ca. 1910 and ca. 1915. Library of Congress Call Number/Physical Location, LC-B2-2940-13 [P&P] LOT 10834 (Corresponding print), Bain News Service photograph collection, Library of Congress Prints and Photographs Division; Digital Id: ggbain 15053 //hdl.loc.gov/loc.pnp/ggbain.15053; Library of Congress Control Number 2014695023; reproduction number LC-DIG-ggbain-15053.

time, John Harvey reported the pertinent nutritional data for all dishes on the San's menu that included percentages of protein, carbohydrates, and fats, as well as the calorie counts.

John Harvey's younger brother Will was no less industrious. Although some would contend that William Keith Kellogg stole his brother's cornflake recipe and empire, that would somewhat misrepresent the case. Will helped develop the cornflake, and it was he that decided added sugar would "sweeten the deal," which infuriated John Harvey. In 1906, Will formed the Battle Creek Toasted Corn Flake Company, which eventually became the Kellogg Company.

In 1916, when his older brother sued for control of the company but lost the case, Will became the controller. Adding sugar to the cornflakes was not Will's only insightful idea. He also created a mixture of oatmeal, wheat, and cornmeal which he baked and dubbed Granula. He managed in addition to create a protein substitute for meat by removing the hulls of peanuts, roasting the peanuts in an oven, and then grinding up the roasted peanuts. He called his new food Nuttose; it was the predecessor of peanut butter.

About 300,000 patients stayed at the San's glassed-in halls and extensive verandas over its 70 plus–year history, and the list of attendees pays tribute to the high-class people drawn into John Harvey Kellogg's promotional flair. Among them were Amelia Earhart, Henry Ford, Harvey Firestone, Warren Harding, Mary Todd Lincoln, James Buick, S. S. Kresge, Montgomery Ward, J. C. Penney, C. W. Post, Johnny Weissmuller, and Edgar Welch. Unfortunately, the San was a victim of the Great Depression; many of the wealthy clientele were no longer able to afford the cost of a stay and it went through several difficult years. It struggled through World War II but then was eventually sold to the army for use as a hospital. The main building still stands and is a federal building.

*   *   *

The legacy of self-help is certainly not lost in the twenty-first century. Gymnasiums, pools, tennis courts, and numerous other sports facilities are testament to the influence that self-help movements in the past had for creating a mindset of preventive health maintenance. Many of the old mineral spring resorts still exist in some form. Daily vitamins are found on shelves in every kind of pharmacy and grocery store, and are a daily part of the breakfast ritual. As Covert Bailey (1991) said in his book *Fit or Fat,* Americans have the most expensive urine in the world.

Whether we take our food supplements in concert with others at health resorts or workshops, and exercise at home with our own equipment or at the club with others, Americans firmly believe that vast segments of their health and well-being can be handled largely on their own. By doing so, we maintain that we can delay the act of crossing the divide to professional medical care longer.

Conclusion

The Road to Wellness

Colonial America was formed by people from radically different traditions, histories, ecologies, and economies. Each of the colonial populations had long traditions of health care, each with unique practices and interpretations, but with shared approaches as well. However, health care in America did not simply originate from the component parts of the colonizers and the colonized, but developed alongside the social, political, and economic endeavors of a developing nation. Thus, one cannot understand the concepts of health and disease without understanding the context in which those concepts were conceived.

Home health care was the only available route for most people early in the colonial process. Experience and knowledge were gained by observation and practice, and consultation with friends and family. Home remedies remained a mainstay for many families and individuals. There were also lay practitioners (midwives, for instance) who had gained experience and knowledge throughout their lifetime; consequently, they were usually those well up in years. Respect for specialists was fundamental, and based on familiarity and reputation.

There were also semiformally trained specialists, such as dentists, apothecaries, and surgeons. They were generally trained through apprenticeships, and were often still bound within the fabric of local knowledge and trust. Many came from the community in which they practiced. Itinerant doctors and dentists moved from place to place providing health care, and they were largely informally trained and not from the immediate communities they served. Finally, formally trained physicians had long practiced in Europe, but their clientele was largely confined to the upper class, aside from itinerant practitioners. They came to America only after an upper class existed.

Consequently, there were multiple layers of health care. Alongside bonded and licensed practitioners were lay practitioners, the latter far less expensive and likely more familiar and trusted. Familiarity was important. It was comfortable, but potentially limited in the care it could provide. Professional help potentially offered more options, but was less familiar. The acceptance of professional practitioners, at least by some and for a limited time, marked the beginning of institutionalized medicine, which came about through a lengthy process and was accompanied by several important developments in American life.

Concepts of specialization in the seventeenth and eighteenth centuries were important contexts for public acceptance of medical specialization. As well, the decline of artisans and emergence of wage labor and specialization were essential for the acceptance of professional, formally trained physicians. Yet, many people could not afford the cost of formally trained physicians. Social class barriers, set within the growing pains of an emerging nation, created immense economic stratification. Poverty and changes in family structure necessitated institutional care for the impoverished, often those without sufficient family ties. Care in the home became something that existed within certain social and economic classes, but not others.

The first half of the nineteenth century was marked by increasing criticism of professional medicine. The hospital infrastructure had serious issues, distrust of formal specialists grew, especially as fueled by the followers of Andrew Jackson, and multiple alternative approaches to health and well-being emerged in the early to mid-1800s. The medical profession, well aware of lax standards of training and the failure of those institutions that had developed, hospitals and almshouses, focused their efforts on licensing and criticisms directed at non–formally trained practitioners.

As the institution of physicians and the infrastructures within which they practiced seemed on the brink of collapse, the Civil War broke out in 1861. Mortality such as witnessed during the Civil War had hardly been seen before, certainly not on American soil at least, and it necessitated understanding and dealing with the inadequacies of American medicine. In four short years, new hospital designs, new approaches to hygiene, and new treatment methods changed the face of American health care. Ambulances, anesthesia, and embalming are but a few of the innovations tied to the Civil War. When America emerged from the war, there were refocused efforts to renovate infrastructure, particularly in urban areas, and bring increased attention to the issues of sanitation and hygiene in water and waste disposal.

New social health movements sprang up for the redesign of the home, for cleanliness both in physical spaces and the body, and for nutrition and wellness. Again, these did not occur in a vacuum. Following the Civil War, America was enveloped in the Industrial Revolution, and social class and economic differences continued to divide the nation. There were those who could avail themselves of new water and sewage systems, of home redesign, of spas and treatment centers, and those who could not.

Yet, slowly, the hygiene movement spread outward, eventually reaching deep into the depths of poverty. In the middle of the nineteenth century, centralized water systems, quarantine, and other innovations began to bring down the mortality rates from infectious disease. Childhood mortality, a major issue prior to about 1850, began to decrease in frequency.

Twentieth-century America saw the increased success of hygiene. With the discovery of pathogens and the acceptance of the germ theory of disease, both in the last quarter of the nineteenth century, hygiene could be targeted differently. Sterilization of physical spaces and medical instruments was an important outcome. As a result, declines in childhood mortality continued, and increased life span took place. Homes and businesses were cleaner and healthier for the most part.

There were exceptions, though. One was the increased use of built environments after 1900, a process that began in the mid-nineteenth century. More and more of people's lives became spent indoors, and sick-building syndrome became one of several problems that were created in built living spaces. A second exception was sexual hygiene. In the post–World War II era, there was a widespread repudiation of the Victorian notion that sexual moderation led to healthy outcomes.

Sex for pleasure, not bound entirely by reproduction, became widely practiced, and women were released from earlier constraints of "proper" behavior. This is not to say that sexually transmitted diseases or promiscuity were not problems earlier—the widespread epidemic of syphilis in the sixteenth century serves as but one example. Rather, it is to say that the means of preventing sexually transmitted diseases and other issues of sexual hygiene were available and became a routine part of the medical profession. However, so did a number of sexually transmitted diseases.

The first half of the twentieth century saw the introduction of antibiotics, new vaccines, and vaccine campaigns, and continued success in meeting the challenges of health and well-being. Our jubilation at the success of institutional medicine continued into the second half of the twentieth century, although home cures and remedies did not disappear. People continued to make decisions about when to seek a medical professional and when to use the old family cures.

It seemed as if infectious disease was well under control, until about 1990. At that time, two major things happened: emerging diseases and antibiotic resistance appeared (Barrett et al. 1998). Both have continued to challenge public health. Especially problematic are new diseases, often tied very closely to ecological impacts. Most are tied to landscape alterations and development, and cross over to humans from other species. The continued alteration of natural habitats has seen continued experiences with new diseases. Some of those new diseases reveal cracks in the American medical system. And so, as America continues to evolve, so do the germs that live with us, and our methods and devotion to hygiene must continue.

Epilogue

It is very strange to complete a book on the growth and history of health and wellness care in America at the exact moment that the entire health system is faced with its most dire moments, and at times seems on the brink of collapse. As I have revised the draft of this book, I've done most of it from Bear Lake, Michigan, where we own our second home. The town is located on one of those wonderful interior northern Michigan lakes, most of them small, peaceful, and restorative.

I walk along the lake many days per year. I grew up near here and this property was the last home of my parents for over 20 years. Here, they ran an antique shop and my Mom raised and sold irises, as well as making doll clothes. They were always eclectic, my folks. I love to be here most of the time, for the slow pace of life, the nature, the familiarity and predictability of many aspects of day to day living.

This year was different. I wrote in Michigan during January, went home to Carrboro, North Carolina, in mid-February, and returned a week later. Lorraine, my lovely wife, joined me here for ten days in mid-March. During that time, the Covid-19 pandemic entered the United States like a high-speed train. Lorraine returned to North Carolina to work, and I remained here alone until mid-June when she returned.

I should perhaps provide some historical context for those who read this years later. In mid- to late 2019, a highly contagious and serious respiratory illness broke out in China. It is often attributed to Wuhan, although that verdict is probably not secure. It raged in China for several months, and then began its expansion beyond the border.

The first cited port of arrival in the United States was in early 2020 in the state of Washington, and it was about that time that public health experts issued calls for action. Unfortunately, the American response was unorganized, chaotic, and largely focused on denial, especially out of the White House of then-president Donald Trump. Daily briefings wove tales of imminent victory over the virus that causes the illness, Covid-19, and of national efforts to produce sufficient personal protective equipment (PPE). State governments were variously left to their own devices to provide PPE for their residents, while at other times subjected to close scrutiny from the federal government.

The medical experts who testified in White House briefings were often shifted on a weekly basis with those supporting a message of hope and victory; clearly, they were the ones who were preferred. In a few short months, America led the world in the number of cases of the disease and of deaths that resulted from it.

I have wondered many times as I recorded my thoughts, what would archaeology, bioarchaeology, and history tell us about the challenges and changes in American health care during this time? Could we possibly reconstruct, a hundred years from now, the precise details of the events in 2020? When I think of the documentary evidence, I wonder, "Could one get a real sense of the honest, factual, representative events that have transpired during the pandemic?" Many times, the accounts conflicted with each other. The messages from the Oval Office certainly contradicted those from various health agencies (CDC, WHO, their own Covid team), resulting in a tapestry of oscillating and often contradictory interpretations and conclusions.

Photographs depict the sudden breakdown of America. Urban centers on fire, broken store windows and looting, cars overturned, and horrible violent death as the ugly head of racism and treatment of the disfranchised captured the eyes and ears of all citizens. There was an unexplained surge of facial masks being worn in almost any setting, and advertising for them overwhelmed the Internet. Yet, peppered within the face mask scenes were those with people in crowded bars and beaches, shoulder to shoulder, arm in arm, dancing, singing, all without face masks.

Archaeological and bioarchaeological data are accumulative by their very nature; but in an environment where accumulation is so rapid, so panic-driven, so overwhelming, how will the resulting material record look decades or centuries from now? What would future interpreters make of the sheer volume of disposable face masks, gloves, test kits, containers, bodies?

Will ventilators be readily apparent for their actual use? And the popular distillery down the road which made highly refined and priced bourbon and vodka—was their sudden switch to manufacturing alcohol sanitizer driven by accounts that using it would provide protection to health and wellness?

Beyond any of my fanciful musings above is the very real observation that we are seeing one of those historic moments when major transitions occur in American health and wellness. If we think about it, we can see the legacy of decades of both growth and stagnation in the methods and institutions for providing health care. We can also see the necessity of rapidly navigating changes required to meet the demands of a novel pathogen, not only through the tools and traditions of health care, but through the behaviors of American (and global) citizens. Sadly, we can also see the resistance on the part of American citizens who cannot accept that they must alter their behaviors in order to provide for adequate health and wellness.

It is somewhat unclear from where I sit at my desk in February of 2021, where this will all progress. America has a new president, Joseph Biden, who is focused on shifting the course of the pandemic. Two vaccines have been developed and are slowly being administered to the public, but the distribution and administration are hampered by a complete absence of organization. A third vaccine is being approved, but the vaccines are coming into the pandemic as several mutations of Covid-19 have been documented. It is clear they are more transmissible, but not clear about whether they are more virulent.

What I do know is that the description of the 1918 influenza pandemic presented in the epilogue of my last book, *Disease and Discrimination* (Hutchinson 2016), is eerily close to our current situation. It is not comforting, except through the knowledge that history and memory are essential to provide lessons and tactics for contemporary events. Please, let us learn just once. Let us recognize that what happened in the past is relevant to what might happen in the present, or in the future. Let us recognize our mistakes, and learn from them.

References Cited

PRIMARY SOURCES

Alcott, William A.
1845   Cold Water Facts. *Water-Cure Journal*, Dec. 15, 21.

Beard, George M.
1881   *American Nervousness, Its Causes and Consequences, A Supplement to Nervous Exhaustion (Neurasthemia)*. New York: G. P. Putnam's Sons.

Beard, George M., and Alphonso D. Rockwell
1871   *A Practical Treatise on the Medicinal and Surgical Uses of Electricity*. New York: William Wood.

Beecher, Catherine E.
1856   *Physiology and Calisthenics for Schools and Families*. New York: Harper and Brothers.

Beecher, Catherine E., and Harriet Beecher Stowe
1971   *The American Woman's Home: Or, Principles of Domestic Science; Being a Guide to the Formation and Maintenance of Economical, Healthful, Beautiful, and Christian Homes*. New York: Arno Press & the New York Times; originally published 1869 by J. B. Ford and Company.

Benezet, Anthony A.
1826   *The Family Physician; Comprising Rules for the Prevention and Cure of Diseases; Calculated Particularly for the Inhabitants of the Western Country, and for Those Who Navigate Its Waters*. Cincinnati, OH: W. H. Woodward.

Biggar, H. P.
1924   *The Voyages of Jacques Cartier*. Ottawa: Acland.

Billings, John Shaw
1870   *A Report on Barracks and Hospitals, with Descriptions of Military Posts*. Circular No. 4. War Department, Surgeon General's Office. Washington, DC: Government Printing Office.

1875a   Hospital Plans. In *Hospital Plans. Five Essays relating to the Construction, Organization & Management of Hospitals, Contributed by their Authors for the Use of the Johns Hopkins Hospital of Baltimore*. New York: William Wood.

1875b   *A Report on the Hygiene of the United States Army, with Descriptions of Military Posts*. Circular No. 8. War Department, Surgeon General's Office. Washington, DC: Government Printing Office.

Brébeuf, Jean de
1636   "Relation of Jean de Brébeuf." *Jesuit Relations* X: 166–169.

Brown, Lawrason, MD
1928   *Rules for Recovery from Pulmonary Tuberculosis.* Philadelphia: Lea & Febiger.

Buchan, William
1772   *Domestic Medicine: or A Treatise on the Prevention and Cure of Diseases,* 2nd edition. Edinburgh: W. Strahan.

1795   *Domestic Medicine: or A Treatise on the Prevention and Cure of Diseases,* 1st American edition. Philadelphia: Thomas Dobson.

1809   *Advice to Mothers, on the Subject of Their Own Health; and of the Means of Promoting the Health, Strength, and Beauty of Their Offspring.* Boston: Joseph Bumstead.

Carey, Matthew
1828   Essays on the Public Charities of Philadelphia. Clark & Raser: Philadephia, 5th edition.

Carter, Landon
1965   *The Diary of Colonel Landon Carter of Sabine Hall, 1752–1778, Volume 1,* edited by Jack P. Greene, pp. 205–206. Richmond: The Virginia Historical Society, William Byrd Press.

Chancellor, C. W., MD
1877   *Report of the Public Charities Reformatories, Prisons and Almshouses, of the State of Maryland.* Frederick, MD: Baughman Brothers. Reprinted in *The State and Public Welfare in Nineteenth-Century America: Five Investigations, 1833–1877,* Gerald Grob, general editor. New York: Arno Press, 1976.

Cooper, Thomas
1824   *A Treatise of Domestic Medicine.* Reading, PA: G. Getz.

Department of Propaganda for Reform
1915   Addison's Galvanic Electric Belt. *Journal of the American Medical Association,* Volume 65, Oct. 2: 1202.

Drake, Daniel
1844   An Introductory Lecture, On the Means of Promoting the Intellectual Improvement of the Students and Physicians of the Valley of the Mississippi. Delivered in the Medical Institute of Louisville, November 4th, 1844. *Medical Examiner and Record of Medical Science* (1844–1853), 03/1845, Volume 8, Issue 3, p. 188.

1850   A Systematic Treatise, Historical, Etiological, and Practical, on the Principal Diseases of the Interior Valley of North America: As They Appear in the Caucasian, African, Indian, and Esquimaux Varieties of Its population. Cincinnati [OH]: W. B. Smith & Co., 1850 [c1849] (Morgan and Overend).

Ely, E. S.
1812   *The Journal of the Stated Preacher to the Hospital and Almshouse, in the City of New York for the Year of Our Lord 1811.* New York: Whiting and Watson.

Ewell, Thomas
1824   *American Family Physician; Detailing Important Means of Preserving Health, from Infancy to Old Age.* Georgetown, DC: J. Thomas.

Formento, Felix
1863   *Notes and Observations on Army Surgery.* New Orleans: L. E. Marchand.
Godey, Louis A.
1859–1887 *Godey's Lady's Book and Magazine.* New York: Godey's Lady's Book Publishing.
Griscom, John H.
1845   *The Sanitary Condition of the Laboring Population of New York, with Suggestions for Improvement.* A discourse delivered on the 30th December 1844, at the Repository of the American Institute. New York: Harper Brothers, 1845. Reprint. New York: Arno Press, 1970.
Gross, S. D.
1862   *A Manual of Military Surgery or Hints on the Emergencies of Field, Camp, and Hospital Practice,* 2nd edition. Philadelphia: J. B. Lippincott & Co.
Gunn, John C.
1830   *Gunn's Domestic Medicine.* Facsimile edition. Knoxville: University of Tennessee Press. Republished 1986.
Hariot, Thomas
1972   *A Brief and True Report of the New Found Land of Virginia.* Reprint. New York: Dover.
Hippocrates of Kos (Hippocrates II)
4th or 5th century BCE   *Airs, Waters, and Places.*
Hitchcock, Edward
1831   *Dyspepsia Forestalled and Resisted, or Lectures on Diet, Regimen, and Employment.* Amherst, MA: J. S. & C. Adams.
Institoris, Henricus (Heinrich Kramer)
1486   *Malleus Maleficarum (Hammer of the Witches).* Originally published in Speyer, Germany.
Jones, John
1776   *Plain concise practical remarks, on the Treatment of Wounds and Fractures; To Which Is Added, An Appendix, On Camp and Military Hospitals; Principally Designed, for the Use of Young Military and Naval Surgeons, in North-America.* Philadelphia: Printed, and sold by Robert Bell, in Third Street, MDCCLXXVI.
Josselyn, John.
1860   New England's Rarities Discovered in Birds, Beasts, Fishes, Serpents, and Plants of That Country. In *Archaeologica Americana, Transactions and Collections of the American Antiquarian Society, Volume IV*, pp. 105–238. Worcester, Mass.: American Antiquarian Society, 1820–1885 (Worcester, Mass. : Printed for the Amarican Society by William Manning).
Kellogg, John Harvey
1876   *The Uses of Water in Health and Disease.* Battle Creek, MI: The Offices of the Health Reformer.
1882   *Household Manual of Domestic Hygiene, Food and Diet.* Battle Creek, MI: Good Health Publishing Company.
1908   *The Battle Creek Sanitarium: History, Organization, Methods.* Battle Creek, MI: Battle Creek Sanitarium.

1913   *Battle Creek Sanitarium: History, Organization, Methods.* Battle Creek, MI: Battle Creek Sanitarium.

Kemble, Frances Anne
1984   *Journal of a Residence on a Georgia Plantation in 1838–1839.* Reprint, edited by John A. Scott; originally published 1863. Athens: University of Georgia Press.

Kirkbride, Thomas Story
1854   *On the Construction, Organization, and General Arrangements of Hospitals for the Insane.* Philadelphia: Lindsay and Blakiston.

Lawson, John
1967   *A New Voyage to Carolina.* Edited & With an Introduction & Notes by Hugh Talmage Lefler. Chapel Hill: University of North Carolina Press; originally published 1709.

Lay, George W.
1910   The Sanitary Privy. *Bulletin North Carolina Board of Health* 25(1): 20–30.

Macfadden, Bernarr
1868–1955   *Physical Culture.* New York: Physical Culture Publishing Co.

Mather, Cotton
1972   *The Angel of Bethesda: An Essay Upon the Common Maladies of Mankind.* Worcester, MA: American Antiquarian Society.

Mathews, William
1848   *A Treatise on Domestic Medicine and Kindred Subjects: Embracing Anatomical and Physiological Sketches of the Human Body.* Indianapolis: J. D. Defrees.

O'Followell, Ludovic
1908   *Le Corset: Histoire—Médecène—Hygiene.* Paris: A. Maloine.

Otis, George A., and D. L. Huntington
1883   Transportation of the Wounded, Chapter XV, pp. 923–982. In *Medical and Surgical History of the War of the Rebellion, Part III, Volume II, Surgical History.* 2nd issue, under the general direction of Joseph K. Barnes. Washington, DC: U.S. Government Printing Office.

Quincy, Josiah
1827   *Report of the Committee Appointed by the Board of Governors of the Poor of the City and Districts of Philadelphia, to Visit the Cities of Baltimore, New-York, Providence, Boston, and Salem.* Philadelphia: Samuel Parker. Reprinted by Rothman, 1971.

Reid, David Boswell
1858   *Ventilation in American Dwellings.* New York: Wiley and Halstead.

Riis, Jacob A.
1890   *How the Other Half Lives: Studies among the Tenements of New York, with illustrations chiefly from photographs taken by the author.* New York: C. Scribner's Sons.

Ruble, Thomas W.
1810   *The American Medical Guide for the Use of Families.* Richmond, KY: E. Harris.

Sharp, Jane
1671   *The Midwives Book: Or the Whole Art of Midwifry Discovered.* London: Simon Miller.

1725   *The Complete Midwife's Companion: or, the Art of Midwifry Improv'd. Directing Child-bearing Women How to Order Themselves in Their Conception, Breeding, Bearing, and Nursing of Children*, 4th edition. London: Simon Miller.

Smith, John
1629   *The General History of Virginia, New England, and the Summer Isles.* . . . Book Four, p. 101. London.

Strachey, William
1610   The True Repertory of the Wreck and Redemption of Sir Thomas Gates, Knight. In *A Voyage to Virginia in 1609*, Louis B. Wright, editor (1965): 1–101.

Stuart, James H.
1864   *A Manual of Free Gymnastic and Dumb-Bell Exercises for the School-Room and Parlor.* Cincinnati, OH: Van Antwerp, Bragg and Company.

Thomson, Samuel
1822   *New Guide to Health or, Botanic Family Physician: Containing a Complete System of Practice, upon a Plan Entirely New, with a Description of the Vegetables Made Use of, and Directions for Preparing and Administering Them to Cure Disease: to Which is Prefixed a Narrative of the Life and Medical Discoveries of the Author.* Boston: Printed for the author by E. G. House.

1824   *Learned Quackery Exposed, or, Theory according to Art: as Exemplified in the Practice of the Fashionable Doctors of the Present Day.* Boston, 1824. 24 pp. Sabin Americana. Gale, Cengage Learning. University of North Carolina at Chapel Hill. July 1, 2018.

U.S. Army Corps of Engineers (USACE)
1864–1865 *Bawdy Houses.* Provost Marshal's Department of Washington, 22nd Army Corps. Record Group 393, Volume 298. Washington, DC: National Archives and Records Administration.

U.S. Department of Commerce
1975   *Historical Statistics of the United States.* Washington, DC: Government Printing Office.

Warner, Amos
1894   *American Charities: A Study in Philanthropy and Economics.* New Brunswick, NJ: Transaction (republished 1989). New York: Thomas Y. Crowell & Co.

Wells, W. R.
1869   *A New Theory of Disease; Based on the Principle That Man Is a Compound Electrical Magnet.* Rochester, NY: C. D. Tracy.

Wesley, John
1764   *Primitive Physick: or, an Easy and Natural Method of Curing Most Diseases,* 12th edition. Philadelphia: A. Steuart.

Woodward, Joseph J.
1871   "The Army Medical Museum at Washington." *Lippincott's Magazine of Popular Literature and Science* 7 (March), pp. 233–242. Washington, DC: J. B. Lippincott and Office of the Librarian of Congress.

Wyatt, Francis
1926   Letter of Sir Francis Wyatt, Governor of Virginia, 1621–1626. *William and Mary Quarterly,* ser: 2, 6 (1926): 117.

SECONDARY SOURCES

Adams, George Worthington
1996   *Doctors in Blue: The Medical History of the Union Army in the Civil War.* Baton Rouge: Louisiana State University Press; originally published in New York: Henry Schuman, 1952.

Allen, Lane
1976   Grandison Harris, Sr.: Slave, Resurrectionist, and Judge. *Bulletin of the Georgia Academy of Science* 34: 192–199.

Anderson, Ann
2000   *Snake Oil, Hustlers and Hambones: The Great American Medicine Show.* Jefferson, NC, and London: McFarland & Company, Inc.

Armstrong, David, and Elizabeth Metzger Armstrong
1991   *The Great American Medicine Show.* New York: Prentice Hall.

Arnold, Paul N.
2009   The Sterilization Controversy. *Cataract and Refractive Surgery Today,* March 2009: 85–86.

Bailey, Covert
1991   *Fit or Fat.* Boston: Mariner Books.

Barrett, R., C. W. Kuzawa, T. McDade, and G. J. Armelagos
1998   Emerging and Re-Emerging Infectious Diseases: The Third Epidemiological Transition. *Annual Reviews of Anthropology* 27: 247–271.

Bearss, E. C.
1970   *Andersonville National Historic Site: Historic Resource Study and Historic Base Map.* Washington, DC: National Park Service, U.S. Department of the Interior.

Bell, Edward L.
1990   The Historical Archaeology of Mortuary Behavior: Coffin Hardware from Uxbridge, Massachusetts. *Historical Archaeology* 24: 54–78.

Benes, Peter
1990   Itinerant Physicians, Healers, and Surgeon-Dentists in New England and New York, 1720–1825. In *Medicine and Healing: The Dublin Seminar for New England Folklife,* edited by Peter Benes and Jane Montague Benes, pp. 95–112. Boston University.

Benes, Peter, and Jane Montague Benes (editors)
1990   *Medicine and Healing: The Dublin Seminar for New England Folklife.* Boston University.

Bengston, Bradley P., and Julian E. Kuz (editors)
1996   *Photographic Atlas of Civil War Injuries: Photographs of Surgical Cases and Specimens Otis Historical Archives.* Grand Rapids, MI: Medical Staff Press.

Berman, Paul
1990   Obstetrical Practice in South Central Massachusetts from 1834 to 1845. In *Medicine and Healing: The Dublin Seminar for New England Folklife,* edited by Peter Benes and Jane Montague Benes, pp. 185–190. Boston University.

Bethard, Wayne
2004   *Lotions, Potions, and Deadly Elixirs: Frontier Medicine in America.* Lanham, MD: Roberts Rinehart [Rowman & Littlefield].

Blake, John
1977   From Buchan to Fishbein: The Literature of Domestic Medicine. In *Medicine without Doctors: Home Health Care in American History,* edited by Guenter B. Risse, Ronald L. Numbers, and Judith Walter Leavitt, pp. 11–30. New York: Science History Publications.

Blakely, Robert L.
1997   A Clandestine Past: Discovery of the Medical College of Georgia and Theoretical Foundations. In *Bones in the Basement: Postmortem Racism in Nineteenth-Century Medical Training,* edited by Robert L. Blakely and Judith M. Harrington, pp. 3–27. Washington, DC: Smithsonian Institution Press.

Blakely, Robert L., and Judith M. Harrington (editors)
1997   *Bones in the Basement: Postmortem Racism in Nineteenth-Century Medical Training.* Washington, DC: Smithsonian Institution Press.

Blakely, Robert L., and Judith M. Harrington
1997   Grave Consequences: The Opportunistic Procurement of Cadavers at the Medical College of Georgia. In *Bones in the Basement: Postmortem Racism in Nineteenth-Century Medical Training,* pp. 162–183. Washington, DC: Smithsonian Institution Press.

Bonasera, Michael C., and Leslie Raymer
2001   Good for What Ails You: Medicinal Use at Five Points. *Historical Archaeology* 35: 49–64.

Boyle, T. Coraghessan
1994   *The Road to Wellville.* New York: Penguin.

Britten, E. H.
1875   *The Electrical Physician: or Self-Cure Through Electricity.* Boston: Dr. William Britten.

Brooks, Stewart
1966   *Civil War Medicine.* Springfield, IL: Charles C. Thomas.

Bush, David R.
2000   Interpreting the Latrines of the Johnson's Island Civil War Military Prison. *Historical Archaeology* 34: 62–78.

Calvert, Karin
1992   *Children in the House: The Material Culture of Early Childhood, 1600–1900.* Boston: Northeastern University Press.

Carnes-MacNaughton, Linda
2016   Mariners Maladies: Examining Medical Equipage from the *Queen Anne's Revenge* Shipwreck. *North Carolina Archaeology* 65: 28–52.

Carnes-MacNaughton, Linda, and Terry M. Harper
2000   The Parity of Privies: Summary Research on Privies in North Carolina. *Historical Archaeology* 34: 97–110.

Casella, Eleanor
2007   *The Archaeology of Institutional Confinement.* Gainesville: University of Florida Press.

Coffin, Margaret M.
1976   *Death in Early America: The History and Folklore of Customs and Superstitions*

of Early Medicine, Funerals, Burials, and Mourning. Nashville, TN: Thomas Nelson.

Cole, Elizabeth
1935 *Fifty Years at the Trudeau Sanatorium: An Historical Sketch in Honor of Its Birthday.* Saranac Lake, NY: Currier Press.

Covey, Herbert C.
2007 *African American Slave Medicine: Herbal and Non-herbal Treatments.* Lanham, MD: Lexington Books.

Crellin, John K., and Jane Philpott
1989 *Herbal Medicine Past and Present, Volume II: A Reference Guide to Medicinal Plants.* Durham, NC: Duke University Press.

Crist, Thomas
2005 Babies in the Privy: Prostitution, Infanticide, and Abortion in New York City's Five Points District. *Historical Archaeology* 39: 19–46.

Crist, Thomas A., Douglas B. Mooney, and Kimberly A. Morrell
2017 "The Mangled Remains of What Had Been Humanity": Evidence of Autopsy and Dissection at Philadelphia's Blockley Almshouse, 1835–1895. In *The Bioarchaeology of Dissection and Autopsy in the United States,* edited by Kenneth C. Nystrom, pp. 259–278. New York: Springer.

Cunningham, H. H.
1958 *Doctors in Gray: The Confederate Medical Service.* Baton Rouge: Louisiana State University Press.

Curry, Leonard P.
1981 *The Free Black in Urban America, 1800–1850: The Shadow of the Dream.* Chicago: University of Chicago Press.

Daniel, T. M.
1997 *Captain of Death: The Story of Tuberculosis.* Rochester, NY: University of Rochester Press.

Decker, William A., MD
2010 *Northern Michigan Asylum: A History of the Traverse City State Hospital.* Traverse City, MI: Arbutus Press.

Demos, John
1970 *A Little Commonwealth: Family Life in Plymouth Colony.* New York: Oxford University Press.

Devine, Shauna
2014 *Learning from the Wounded: The Civil War and the Rise of American Medical Science.* Chapel Hill: University of North Carolina Press.

Dougherty, Sean P., and Norman C. Sullivan
2017 Autopsy, Dissection, and Anatomical Exploration: The Postmortem Fate of the Underclass and Institutionalized in Old Milwaukee. In *The Bioarchaeology of Dissection and Autopsy in the United States,* edited by Kenneth C. Nystrom, pp. 205–236. New York: Springer.

Dubos, René, and Jean Dubos
1996 *The White Plague: Tuberculosis, Man, and Society.* New Brunswick, NJ: Rutgers University Press.

Duffy, John
1968   *A History of Public Health in New York City 1625–1866.* New York: Russell Sage Foundation.
1993   *From Humors to Medical Science: A History of American Medicine,* 2nd edition. Urbana and Chicago: University of Illinois Press.

Duncan, Neil A.
1997   Bottles in the Basement: Artifactual Evidence of Late Nineteenth-Century Health Care from the Medical College of Georgia. In *Bones in the Basement: Postmortem Racism in Nineteenth-Century Medical Training,* edited by Robert L. Blakely and Judith M. Harrington, pp. 48–80. Washington, DC: Smithsonian Institution Press.

Ferguson, Leland
1992   *Uncommon Ground: Archaeology and Early African America, 1650–1800.* Washington, DC: Smithsonian Institution Press.
1999   "The Cross Is a Magic Sign": Marks on Eighteenth-Century Bowls from South Carolina. In *"I, Too, Am America": Archaeological Studies of African-American Life,* edited by Theresa A. Singleton, pp. 116–131. Charlottesville: University Press of Virginia.

Ferguson, Leland, and Kelly Goldberg
2019   From the Earth: Spirituality, Medicine Vessels, and Consecrated Bowls as Responses to Slavery in the South Carolina Lowcountry. *Journal of African Diaspora Archaeology and Heritage,* DOI:10.1080/21619441.2019.1690843.

Fett, Sharla
2002   *Working Cures: Healing, Health, and Power on Southern Slave Plantations.* Chapel Hill: University of North Carolina Press.

Figg, Laurann, and Jane Farrell-Beck
1993   Amputation in the Civil War: Physical and Social Dimensions. *Journal of the History of Medicine and Allied Sciences* 48: 454–475.

Fisher, Charles L., Karl J. Reinhard, Matthew Kirk, and Justin DiVirgilio
2007   Privies and Parasites: The Archaeology of Health Conditions in Albany, New York. *Historical Archaeology* 41: 172–197.

Flannery, Michael A.
2017   *Civil War Pharmacy: A History,* 2nd edition. Carbondale: Southern Illinois University Press.

Fox, Anne A., and Cheryl Lynn Highley
1985   *History and Archaeology of the Hot Wells Hotel Site, 41 BX 237.* Center for Archaeological Research, The University of Texas at San Antonio, Archaeological Survey Report No. 152.

Freeman, Frank R.
2001   *Gangrene and Glory: Medical Care during the American Civil War.* Urbana: University of Illinois Press.

Gallos, Philip L.
1985   *Cure Cottages of Saranac Lake: Architecture and History of a Pioneer Health Resort.* Saranac Lake, NY: Historic Saranac Lake.

Gilfoyle, Timothy J.
1992   *City of Eros: New York City, Prostitution, and the Commercialization of Sex, 1790–1920.* New York: Norton.
Gill, Harold B.
1972   *The Apothecary in Colonial Virginia.* Williamsburg Foundation; distributed by the University Press of Virginia, Charlottesville.
Grauer, Anne L., and Elizabeth M. McNamara
1995   A Piece of Chicago's Past: Exploring Childhood Mortality in the Dunning Poorhouse Cemetary. In Anne L. Grauer (editor), *Bodies of Evidence: Reconstructing History through Skeletal Analysis*, pp. 91–103. New York: Wiley-Liss.
Grauer, Anne L., Elizabeth M. McNamara, and Diane Houdek
1998   A History of Their Own: Patterns of Death in a Nineteenth-Century Poorhouse. In Anne L. Grauer and Patty Stuart-Macadam (editors), Sex and Gender in Paleopathological Perspective, pp. 149–164. Cambridge: Cambridge University Press.
Grauer, Anne L., Laura A. Williams, and M. Catherine Bird
2016   Life and Death in Nineteenth-Century Peoria, Illinois: Taking a Biocultural Approach to Understanding the Past. In *New Directions in Biocultural Anthropology*, edited by Molly K. Zuckerman and Debra L. Martin, pp. 201–217. New York: John Wiley & Sons.
Grauer, Anne L., Vanessa Lathrop, and Taylor Timoteo
2017   Exploring Evidence of Nineteenth Century Dissection in the Dunning Poorhouse Cemetery. In *The Bioarchaeology of Dissection and Autopsy in the United States,* edited by Kenneth C. Nystrom, pp. 301–314. New York: Springer.
Green, Harvey
1986   *Fit For America: Health, Fitness, Sport, and American Society.* New York: Pantheon Books.
Grob, Gerald N.
1973   *Mental Institutions in America: Social Policy to 1875.* New York: The Free Press.
1994   *The Mad Among Us: A History of the Care of America's Mentally Ill.* New York and Toronto: The Free Press.
Hacker, J. David
2011   A Census Based Account of the Civil War Dead. *Civil War History* 57: 307–348.
Haines, Michael R.
1998   Estimated Life Tables for the United States, 1850–1910. *Historical Methods* 31: 149–169.
Hallowell, A. I.
1935   The Bulbed Enema Syringe in North America. *American Anthropologist* 37: 708–710.
Harrington, Judith M.
1997   Death and Disease: The Paleopathology of the Medical College of Georgia Cadaver Sample. In *Bones in the Basement: Postmortem Racism in Nineteenth-Century Medical Training,* edited by Robert L. Blakely and Judith M. Harrington, pp. 261–311. Washington, DC: Smithsonian Institution Press.

Heck, Dana B., and Joseph Balicki
1998   Katherine Naylor's "House of Office": A Seventeenth-Century Privy. *Historical Archaeology* 32: 24–37.
Hesseltine, William B.
1930   *Civil War Prisons.* Columbus: Ohio State University Press.
Higgins, Roseanne L., and Joyce E. Sirianni
1995   An Assessment of Health and Mortality of Nineteenth Century Rochester, New York Using Historic Records and the Highland Park Skeletal Collection. In *Bodies of Evidence: Reconstructing History through Skeletal Analysis,* edited by Anne L. Grauer, pp. 121–136. New York: John Wiley and Sons.
Higgins, Rosanne L., Michael R. Haines, Lorena Walsh, and Joyce E. Sirianni
2002   The Poor in the Mid-Nineteenth Century Northeastern United States: Evidence from the Monroe County Almshouse, Rochester, New York. In *The Backbone of History: Health and Nutrition in the Western Hemisphere,* edited by Richard Steckel and Jerome C. Rose, pp. 162–184. Cambridge: Cambridge University Press.
Hill, Marilynn W.
1993   *Their Sister's Keepers: Prostitution in New York City, 1830–1870.* Berkeley: University of California Press.
Hillson, Simon
1996   *Dental Anthropology.* London: Cambridge University Press.
Historic Alexandria
2018   Archaeology at the Stabler-Leadbeater Apothecary Shop. www.alexandriava.gov/uploadedFiles/historic/info/archaeology/HistoricStructuresReportMorton1984Apothecary.pdf
Hodge, Christina J., Jane Lyden Rousseau, and Michèle E. Morgan
2017   Teachings of the Dead: The Archaeology of Anatomized Remains from Holden Chapel, Harvard University. In *The Bioarchaeology of Dissection and Autopsy in the United States,* edited by Kenneth C. Nystrom, pp. 115–142. New York: Springer.
Hodge, Hugh Lenox
1866   *The Principles and Practice of Obstetrics.* Philadelphia: Henry C. Lea.
Howson, Jean E.
1993   The Archaeology of 19th-Century Health and Hygiene at the Sullivan Street Site, New York City. *Northeast Historical Archaeology* 22 (1): 137–160.
Hubbard, Mercer Reeves (editor)
1998   *The Country Doctor Museum,* 3rd edition. Bailey, NC: The Country Doctor Museum.
Humphrey, David C.
1973   Dissection and Discrimination: The Social Origins of Cadavers in America, 1760–1915. *Bulletin of the New York Academy of Medicine* 49: 819–827.
Humphreys, Margaret
2013   *Marrow of Tragedy: The Health Crisis of the American Civil War.* Baltimore: Johns Hopkins University Press.

Hunkin, Tim
2004 *Dr. Graham's Celestial Bed at the Temple of Hymen, Pall Mall, Anno Domini 1782*, http://www.timhunkin.com/a108_celestial_bed.htm.

Hutchinson, Dale L.
2016 *Disease and Discrimination: Poverty and Pestilence in Colonial Atlantic America.* Gainesville: University Press of Florida.

Hyatt, Harry M.
1970 *Hoodoo-Conjuration-Witchcraft-Rootwork, Volume 1.* St. Louis, MO: Harry Middleton Hyatt.

Jackson, Harold
1997 Race and the Politics of Medicine in Nineteenth-Century Georgia. In *Bones in the Basement: Postmortem Racism in Nineteenth-Century Medical Training*, edited by Robert L. Blakely and Judith M. Harrington, pp. 184–205. Washington, DC: Smithsonian Institution Press.

Johnson, Heidi
2001 *Angels in the Architecture: A Photographic Essay to an American Asylum.* Detroit, MI: Wayne State University Press.

Katz, Michael B.
1986 *In the Shadow of the Poorhouse: A Social History of Welfare in America.* New York: Basic Books.

Kesey, Ken
1970 *One Flew Over the Cuckoo's Nest.* New York: Viking.

King, John
1870 *The American Dispensatory*, 8th edition. Cincinnati, OH: Wilstach, Baldwin, and Company.

Kleinberg, S .J.
1977 Death and the Working Class. *Journal of Popular Culture* 11.1: 193–209.

Klepp, Susan E.
1994 Lost, Hidden, Obstructed, and Repressed: Contraceptive and Abortive Technology in the Early Delaware Valley. In *Early American Technology: Making and Doing Things from the Colonial Era to 1850,* edited by Judith A. McGaw, pp. 68–113. Chapel Hill: University of North Carolina Press.

Krochmal, Arnold, and Connie Krochmal
1973 *A Guide to the Medicinal Plants of the United States.* New York: Quadrangle/The New York Times Book Company.

Krogman, Wilton Marion, and M. Yaşar İşcan
1986 *The Human Skeleton in Forensic Medicine,* 2nd edition. Springfield, IL: Charles C. Thomas.

Kuz, Julian E., and Bradley P. Bengtson
1996 *Orthopedic Injuries of the Civil War: An Atlas of Orthopedic Injuries and Treatments during the Civil War.* Kennesaw, GA: Kennesaw Mountain Press.

Lane, Roger
1997 *Murder in America: A History.* Columbus: Ohio State University Press.

Larson, Lewis H., and Morgan R. Crook
1975 An Archeological [*sic*] Investigation at Andersonville National Historic Site,

Sumter and Macon Counties, Georgia. Unpublished Report. Tallahassee: Southeast Archaeological Center, National Park Service.

Last, John M.
2001   Miasma Theory. In *Encyclopedia of Public Health,* edited by Lester Breslow, pp. 765–766. New York: Macmillan Reference.

Leavitt, Judith W.
1986   *Brought to Bed: Childbearing in America, 1750–1950.* New York: Oxford University Press.

Lewis, Dio
1862   *The New Gymnastics for Men, Women, and Children.* Boston: Ticknor and Fields

Logan, O.
1989   *Motherwit: An Alabama Midwife's Story.* New York: E. P. Dutton.

Lusingnan, Kim
2004   A Historical and Osteological Analysis of Postmortem Medical Practices from the Albany County Almshouse Cemetery Skeletal Sample. M.A. thesis, Department of Anthropology, State University of New York at Albany.

Lusingnan Lowe, Kim
2017   A Historical and Osteological Analysis of Postmortem Medical Practices from the Albany County Almshouse Cemetery Skeletal Sample in Albany, New York. In *The Bioarchaeology of Dissection and Autopsy in the United States,* edited by Kenneth C. Nystrom, pp. 315–334. New York: Springer.

Lyons, Clare A.
2006   *Sex among the Rabble: An Intimate History of Gender and Power in the Age of Revolution.* Chapel Hill: University of North Carolina Press.

Mann, Robert W., Douglas W. Owsley and Paul A. Shackel
1991   A Reconstruction of 19th-Century Surgical Techniques: Bones in Dr. Thompson's Privy. *Historical Archaeology* 25: 106–112.

Mathews, Holly M.
1992a   Doctors and Root Doctors: Patients Who Use Both. In *Herbal and Magical Medicine: Traditional Healing Today,* edited by James Kirkland, Holly Mathews, Charles W. Sullivan III, and Karen Baldwin, pp. 68–98. Durham, NC: Duke University Press.
1992b   Killing the Medical Self-Help Tradition among African Americans: The Case of Lay Midwifery in North Carolina, 1912–1983. In *African Americans in the South,* edited by Hans Baer and Yvonne Jones, pp. 60–78. Athens: University of Georgia Press.

McFarlin, Shannon C., and Lawrence E. Wineski
1997   The Cutting Edge: Experimental Anatomy and the Reconstruction of Nineteenth-Century Dissection Techniques. In *Bones in the Basement: Postmortem Racism in Nineteenth-Century Medical Training,* edited by Robert L. Blakely and Judith M. Harrington, pp. 107–161. Washington, DC: Smithsonian Institution Press.

Mehta, Jayur
2007   A Study of Sweat Lodges in the Southeastern United States. M.A. thesis, University of Alabama–Tuscaloosa.

Miller, Chris
2005   *Traverse City State Hospital.* Charleston: Arcadia Publishing.
Mongeau, B.
1985   The "Granny" Midwives: A Study of a Folk Institution in the Process of Social Disintegration. PhD dissertation, Department of Sociology, University of North Carolina–Chapel Hill.
Mrozowski, S. A., E. L. Bell, Mary C. Beaudry, D. B. Landon, and G. K. Kelso
1989   Living on the Boott: Health and Wellbeing in a Boardinghouse Population. *World Archaeology* 21: 298–319.
Munsey, Cecil
2003   Lydia's Medicine: 130 Years Later. https://www.fohbc.org/PDF_Files/Pinkham_130YrsLater.pdf.
Murphy, Shirley F. (editor)
1883   *Our Homes.* London: Cassell.
Murray, John F., Dean E. Schraufnagel, and Philip C. Hopewell
2015   Treatment of Tuberculosis: A Historical Perspective. *Annals of the American Thoracic Society* 12(12): 1749–1759.
National Public Radio (NPR)
2018   Interview with Vanessa Gamble on *All Things Considered*, 5:10 p.m.
New York State Select Committee Appointed to Visit Charitable Institutions Supported by the State
1857   *Report of Select Committee Appointed to Visit Charitable Institutions Supported by the State, and all City and County Poor and Work Houses and Jails.* Reprinted in *The State and Public Welfare in Nineteenth-Century America: Five Investigations, 1833–1877*, Gerald Grob, general editor. New York: Arno Press, 1976.
Nystrom, Kenneth C.
2011   Postmortem Examinations and the Embodiment of Inequality in 19th Century United States. *International Journal of Paleopathology* 1: 164–172.
2014   The Bioarchaeology of Structural Violence and Dissection in the 19th Century United States. *American Anthropologist* 116: 765–779.
Nystrom, Kenneth C. (editor)
2017   *The Bioarchaeology of Dissection and Autopsy in the United States.* New York: Springer.
Nystrom, Kenneth C., Joyce Sirianni, Rosanne Higgins, Douglas Perrelli, and Jennifer L. Liber Raines
2017   Structural Inequality and Postmortem Examination at the Erie County Poorhouse. In *The Bioarchaeology of Dissection and Autopsy in the United States*, edited by Kenneth C. Nystrom, pp. 279–300. New York: Springer.
Olson, Randall J.
2009   Single-Use Instruments. *Cataract and Refractive Surgery Today*, March 2009: 84, 87.
Ortner, Donald J.
2003   *Identification of Pathological Conditions in Human Skeletal Remains*, 2nd edition. San Diego, CA: Academic Press.

Owsley, Douglas W., Karin S. Bruwelheide, Richard L. Jantz, Jodi L. Koste, and Merry Outlaw
2017   Skeletal Evidence of Anatomical and Surgical Training in Nineteenth-Century Richmond. In *The Bioarchaeology of Dissection and Autopsy in the United States*, edited by Kenneth C. Nystrom, pp. 143–164. New York: Springer.

Parks, Amanda L.
2018   The Semi-Subterranean Sweat Lodges of the Redeemer Site. M.A. thesis, University of Western Ontario, London, Ontario.

Parramore, Thomas
1971   The Country Doctor. Address Given at the Dedication of the Country Doctor Museum. In *The Country Doctor Museum*, edited by Mercer Reeves Hubbard, pp. 9–14. Bailey, NC: The Country Doctor Museum.

Plath, Sylvia
1971   *The Bell Jar.* New York: Harper and Row.

Prentice, Guy, and Marie C. Prentice
2000   Far from the Battlefield: Archaeology at Anderson Prison. In *Archaeological Perspectives on the Civil War*, edited by Clarence R. Geier and Stephen R. Potter, pp. 166–187. Gainesville: University of Florida Press.

Reinhard, Karl J.
2000   Parasitic Disease at Five Points: Parasitological Analysis of Sediments from the Courthouse Block. In *Tales of Five Points: Working-Class Life in Nineteenth-Century New York, Volume II, An Interpretive Approach to Understanding Working-Class Life*, edited by Rebecca Yamin, pp. 391–404. West Chester, PA: John Milner Associates.

Rhode, Michael
1996   Foreword. In *Photographic Atlas of Civil War Injuries: Photographs of Surgical Cases and Specimens Otis Historical Archives*, edited by Bradley P. Bengston and Julian E. Kuz, p. vi. Grand Rapids, MI: Medical Staff Press.

Richardson, Ruth
1987   *Death, Dissection and the Destitute.* London: Routledge and Kegan Paul.

Riddle, John M.
1997   *Eve's Herbs: A History of Conception and Abortion in the West.* Cambridge: Harvard University Press.

Risse, Guenter B.
1977   Introduction. In *Medicine without Doctors: Home Health Care in American History*, edited by Guenter B. Risse, Ronald L. Numbers, and Judith Walter Leavitt, pp. 1–9. New York: Science History Publications.

Risse, Guenter B., Ronald L. Numbers, and Judith Walter Leavitt (editors)
1977   *Medicine without Doctors: Home Health Care in American History.* New York: Science History Publications.

Roberts, Charlotte A., and Jane E. Buikstra
2003   *The Bioarchaeology of Tuberculosis: A Global View on a Reemerging Disease.* Gainesville: University Press of Florida.

Rosenberg, Charles
1987   *The Care of Strangers: The Rise of America's Hospital System.* New York: Basic Books.

Rothman, David J.
1971   *Poverty, U.S.A., The Historical Record: The Almshouse Experience, Collected Reports.* New York: Arno Press & The New York Times.
2002   *The Discovery of the Asylum: Social Order and Disorder in the New Republic,* revised edition. New York: Aldine de Gruyter.

Rothschild, Nan A., and Diana DiZerega Wall
2014   *The Archaeology of American Cities.* Gainesville: University of Florida Press.

Sappol, Michael
2002   *A Traffic of Dead Bodies: Anatomy and Embodied Social Identity in Nineteenth-Century America.* Princeton, NJ: Princeton University Press.

Savitt, Todd L.
1982   The Use of Blacks for Medical Experimentation and Demonstration in the American South. *Journal of Southern History* 48: 331–348.
1990   *Fevers, Agues, and Cures: Medical Life in Old Virginia.* Richmond: The Virginia Historical Society.

Schultz, Jane
2004   *Women at the Front: Hospital Workers in Civil War America.* Chapel Hill: University of North Carolina Press.

Schwartz, Marie Jenkins
2006   *Birthing a Slave: Motherhood and Medicine in the American South.* Cambridge:: Harvard University Press.

Seifert, Donna J., and Joseph Balicki
2005   Mary Ann Hall's House. *Historical Archaeology* 39 (1): 59–73.

Steele, Earle, and Kristen M. Hains
2001   *Beauty Is Therapy: Memories of the Traverse City State Hospital.* Traverse City, MI: Denali and Company.

Steele, Volney
2005   *Bleed, Blister & Purge: A History of Medicine on the American Frontier.* Missoula, MT: Mountain Press.

Stohler, Jacob
1996   Outhouses Left Out of State's Progress. *Raleigh News and Observer,* 3 September: A1, A9. Raleigh, NC.

Stone, Paul
2011   *Legacy of Excellence: The Armed Forces Institute of Pathology, 1862–2011.* Published by the Borden Institute, U.S. Army Medical Department, Fort Detrick, Maryland, & Fort Sam Houston, Texas, for sale by the Superintendent of Documents, U.S. Government Printing Office.

Sutter, Richard C.
1995   Dental Pathologies among Inmates of the Monroe County Poorhouse. In *Bodies of Evidence: Reconstructing History through Skeletal Analysis,* edited by Anne L. Grauer, pp. 185–196. New York: John Wiley and Sons.

Tannenbaum, Rebecca
2002   *The Healer's Calling: Women and Medicine in Early New England.* Ithaca: Cornell University Press.
2012   *Health and Wellness in Colonial America.* Santa Barbara, CA: Greenwood Press.

Tedlock, Dennis, and Barbara Tedlock (editors)
1975   *Teachings from the American Earth: Indian Religion and Philosophy.* New York: Liveright.

Thompson, John D., and Grace Goldin
1975   *The Hospital: A Social and Architectural History.* New Haven and London: Yale University Press.

Thoms, Alston V.
2004   Sand Blows Desperately: Land-Use History and Site Integrity at Camp Ford, a Confederate POW Camp in East Texas. *Historical Archaeology* 38: 73–95.

Toledo-Pereyra, Luis H.
2006   *A History of American Medicine from the Colonial Period to the Early Twentieth Century.* Lewiston, NY: The Edwin Mellen Press.

Tomes, Nancy
2001   Introduction. In *Angels in the Architecture: A Photographic Elegy to an American Asylum,* by Heidi Johnson. Detroit, MI: Wayne State University Press.

U.S. Department of Labor Statistics
2020   Currency Calculator. https://www.bls.gov/data/inflation_calculator.htm.

Veit, Richard
1996   "A Ray of Sunshine in the Sickroom": Archaeological Insights into Late 19th- and Early 20th-Century Medicine and Anesthesia. *Northeast Historical Archaeology* 25: 33–50.

Vesalius, Andreas
1543   *De Humani corporis fabrica libri septem.* Basil: Ex officina I. Operini.

Vogel, Virgil J.
1970   *American Indian Medicine.* Norman: University of Oklahoma Press.

Wagner, David
2005   *The Poorhouse: America's Forgotten Institution.* Lanham, MD: Rowman & Littlefield.

Walker, Philip, R. R. Bathhurst, Rebecca Richman, T. Gjerdrum, and Valerie Andrushko
2009   The Causes of Porotic Hyperostosis and Cribra Orbitalia: A Reappraisal of the Iron-Deficiency Anemia Hypothesis. *American Journal of Physical Anthropology* 139(2): 109–125.

Wall, L. L.
2006   The Medical Ethics of Dr. J. Marion Sims: A Fresh Look at the Historical Record. *Journal of Medical Ethics* 32: 346–350.

Watson, Patricia A.
1991   *The Angelical Conjunction: The Preacher-Physicians of Colonial New England.* Knoxville: University of Tennessee Press.

Weinberger, Bernard
1948   *An Introduction to the History of Dentistry in America,* two volumes. St. Louis, MO: Mosby.

Weiss, Harry B., and Howard R. Kemble
1962   *They Took to the Waters: The Forgotten Mineral Springs of New Jersey and Nearby Pennsylvania and Delaware.* Trenton, NJ: The Past Times Press.
Wigglesworth, William C.
1980   Surgery in Massachusetts, 1620–1800. In *Medicine in Colonial Massachusetts, 1620–1820,* edited by the Colonial Society of Massachusetts, pp. 215–246. Charlottesville: University Press of Virginia.
Wilde-Ramsing, Mark U., and Linda F. Carnes-McNaughton
2018   *Blackbeard's Sunken Prize: The 300-Year Voyage of* Queen Anne's Revenge. Chapel Hill, NC: Univeristy of North Carolina Press.
Wilkie, Laurie A.
2003   *The Archaeology of Mothering: An African-American Midwife's Tale.* New York: Routledge.
Williams, William H.
1976   *America's First Hospital: The Pennsylvania Hospital: 1751–1841.* Wayne, PA: Haverford House Publishers.
Wood, Marilynn H.
1993   *Their Sister's Keeper: Prostitution in New York City 1830–1870.* Berkeley: University of California Press.
Yamin, Rebecca
1998   Lurid Tales and Homely Stories of New York's Notorious Five Points. *Historical Archaeology* 32: 74–85.
2000   *Tales of Five Points: Working-Class Life in Nineteenth-Century New York,* six volumes. Prepared for Edwards and Kelcy Engineers, Inc., and General Services Administration, Region 2. John Milner Associates (now Commonwealth Heritage Group, Inc.), 535 North Church Street, West Chester, Pennsylvania.
2005   Wealthy, Free, and Female: Prostitution in Nineteenth-Century New York. *Historical Archaeology* 39: 4–18.
Yamin, Rebecca, and Donna J. Seifert
2019   *The Archaeology of Prostitution and Clandestine Pursuits.* Gainesville: University of Florida Press.
Young, James Harvey
1961   *The Toadstool Millionaires: A Social History of Patent Medicines in America before Federal Regulation.* Princeton, NJ: Princeton University Press.
1977   Patent Medicines and the Self-Help Syndrome. In *Medicine without Doctors: Home Health Care in American History,* edited by Guenter B. Risse, Ronald L. Numbers, and Judith Walter Leavitt, pp. 95–116. New York: Science History Publications.
Zwelling, Shomer S.
1985   *Quest for a Cure: The Public Hospital in Williamsburg, Virginia, 1773–1885.* Williamsburg, VA: Colonial Williamsburg Foundation.

Index

Page numbers in *italics* refer to illustrations.

Abortifacients, 30
Abortion, 35, 54–55, 163–65
Adams, Samuel Hopkins, 162
Adirondack Recliner, 144
Advent Review and Sabbath Herald, 169
Advertising, for patent medicines, 151, 153
African health care traditions: blended with European and Native American traditions, 2, 4–5; on cause of disease, 17; elder enslaved women, 17; faith and healing, 16–17; handling of corpses, 71–72; treatments for disease, 17–19; women's health care, 30
Airs, Waters, and Places (Hippocrates), 20
Alcott, Dr. William, 86, 88, 168, 176
Algonkian people, 16
Allcock's Porous Plasters, 153
Allopathic medicine, criticism of, 88–91
Almshouses, 50, 55–61, 74–77
Aloe *(Aloe barbadensis),* 29
Ambulance transport, 103
Amenorrhea, 29
American Dispensatory (King), 151
American Family Physician (Ewell), 31
American Hydropathic Institute, 171
American Indians. *See* Native American health care traditions; *names of individual tribes*
American Medical Association (AMA), 88–89, 165
The American Medical Guide for the Use of Families (Ruble), 31
American Nervousness (Beard), 172–73
American Woman's Home (Beecher), 176
Amputation, 105–10, *109*
Anatomical dissection, 77–81
Anatomy, training in, 68, 73, 114. *See also* Dead body trade
Anatomy Acts, 72–73, 76, 80
Ancestry determination, of skeletal remains, 77
Andersonville prison, 110–12
Anemia, 58
Anesthesia, 91–92, 93–94, 106, *107*
The Angel of Bethesda (Mather), 36
Animal waste. *See* Hygiene, public
Antibiotic resistance, 186
Antibiotics, 144
Apache people, 15
Apothecaries, 37–38; apothecary shops, 154–59; contrasted with physicians, 155, 161–62; equipment, 155–56
Archaeological sites: Albany, New York, sewer system, 121; Albany County Almshouse, 75; Andersonville prison, 110–12; Cooper River, South Carolina, 19; Erie County Poorhouse, 75–76; Greenwich Village, Sullivan Street privies, 120; Highland Park Skeletal Collection, 60; Holden Chapel, Harvard Medical School, 80; Hot Wells Hotel, 173–74; Johnson's Island, 112; Katherine Naylor's house, Boston, 119–20; Medical College of Georgia, 78–79, 154; Medical College of Virginia, 79; Monroe County Poorhouse, 59–60; New Brunswick, New Jersey, 91–94, 106;

210 · Index

Archaeological sites—*continued*
   New York, Five Points District, 120–21; New York City brothels, 52–54; Peoria City Cemetery, 60–61; Perryman house, Mobile, Alabama, 165–66; Philadelphia Almshouse, 76; privies, 118–19; *Queen Anne's Revenge (QAR)*, 48–49; Redeemer site, Smiley Rock and Poplar Cove, 14; Stabler-Leadbeater shop, 159; Uxbridge Almshouse, 69; Washington, DC, brothels, 51–52
Archaeology: bias and accuracy of sources, 3–4; and postmortem disfiguration, 73–74
Architecture: asylum design, 137–39; hospital design, 131, 133; pavilion hospital design, 99–101, *100*, 131, 133, 145
Armed Forces Institute of Pathology (AFIP), 112–13
Armed Forces Medical Museum, 112
Army Medical Museum, 112–13
Asafetida (*Ferula* sp.), 19, 30
Astringents, 15, 152
Asylums for special needs patients, 135–41; asylum design, 137–39
Atlas, Charles, 178
Author: childhood experiences in family pharmacy, 1; sources utilized, 2–3
Autopsies, 74
Ayer's Cathartic Pills, 153

Bacteriology. *See* Germ theory
Bailey, Covert, 181
Baker, John, 39
Bakongo ritual, 19
Bard, John, 66
Barnes, Joseph K., 110
Barnes' Magnolia Water, 154
Barton, Clara, 104
Bathing and personal hygiene, 129
Battle Creek Sanitarium, 7, 178–81, *180*
Battlefield medicine during Civil war, 103–5
Battlefield transport, 103
Battle of Bull Run, 103
Battle of Gettysburg, 105
Battle of Shiloh, 98

Bayberries (*Myrica* sp.), 15, 152
Bearberry (*Arctostaphylus uva ursi*), 16
Beard, George M., 172–73
"Beautiful therapy" for mental health, 137–40
Beds and hygiene, 128–29
Beecher, Catherine, 88, 176
Beef tapeworms (*Taenia saginata*), 119, 121
Bell, William, 109
The Bell Jar (Plath), 141
Benes, Peter, 38
Benezet, Anthony A., 31
Beriberi, 169
Bernhardt, Sarah, 174
Biden, Joseph, 189
Bigelow, Charles, 160
Billings, John Shaw, 110, 113, 132–33
The Bioarchaeology of Dissection and Autopsy in the U.S., 74–75
Birth, 28, 50. *See also* Midwives
Birth control, 92, 164. *See also* Emmenagogues
Birthing stools, 33–34
Bitters, 153
Blackbeard, 48
Black bile, in humoural theory, 20
Blakely, Robert L., 78
Blistering, 84
Blood, in humoural theory, 20
Bloodletting, 21, 84, 85
Body snatchers, 69–70
Boneset (*Eupatorium perperfoliatum*), 16, 152
Boott Cotton Mills Corporation, 122–23
Botanical medicines, 87–88, 152. *See also specific plant names*
Boyle, T. Coraghessan, 179
Boylston, Zabdiel, 37, 155
Breakfast cereal, 179, 180–81
Breastfeeding, 26–27
Brébeuf, Father Jean de, 13
Broderick, Matthew, 179
Brothels, 50–55, 120–21
Brown, Dr. Lawrason, 143–44
Brown's Vegetable Cure for Female Weakness, 164
Buchan, William, 30–31

Buick, James, 181
Burial: of cadavers, 73–74; and Christian beliefs, 68

Cadavers, trade in, 68–73
Calomel (mercurous chloride), 84–85, 87, 108, 110
Camphor, 85
Cantharides (Spanish fly), 84–85
Capsicum (*Capsicum* sp.), 24
Carbolic acid, 132
Carey, Matthew, 46
Carnes-McNaughton, Linda, 49
Carter, Landon, 37
Carter's Little Liver Pills, 153
Cartier, Jacques, 169
Cathartics, 15, 152
Celestial Bed, 38–39
Cereal, breakfast, 179, 180–81
Cesspits, 116–17, 124
Chamberland, Charles, 134
Chancellor, C. W., 134–35
Cherokee people, 12, 15, 16
Cherry, wild *(Prunus avium)*, 15
Chewing (Fletcherization), 169
Childbirth, 28, 50. See also Midwives
Childhood mortality, 28
Children, care of, 26–28
Chimborazo Hospital, 103
Chloroform, 93, 106
Cholera, 125
Christianity: and burial of bodies, 68; and healing practices, 20
Cinchona (*Chinchona* sp.), 16
Civil War: Andersonville prison, 110–12; anesthesia use, 93–94; Army Medical Museum, 112–13; battlefield medicine, 103–5; Battle of Bull Run, 103; Battle of Gettysburg, 105; Battle of Shiloh, 98; hospitals, 99–103; and infectious disease, 98, 104; influence on medicine, 6, 97–99, 184–85; Johnson's Island, 112; and medical reformation, 98–99; prisoners of war, 110–12; surgery and amputation, 105–10
Coca-Cola, 7
Cod liver oil, 154
Cody, Buffalo Bill, 160

Colonoware bowls, *18*, 19
Commodes, 126, *127*
Comstock Act (1873), 164
Conception, early ideas concerning, 29
Consumption (tuberculosis), 128, 142–45
Contraception, 92, 164. See also Emmenagogues
Control and Prevention of Infectious Diseases, 107
Cooper, Thomas, 31
Cornflakes, 179, 180
Corsets, 176, *177*
Country Doctor Museum, 90
Covid-19 pandemic, 48, 187–89
Cradleboards, 27
Cradles, 28
Creek people, 15
Croton Aqueduct, 123–24
Cyclical nature of universe, 12

Davice, William, 155
Dead body trade, 68–73
Death records, 57–58, 61
Deficiency diseases: beriberi, 169; in Civil War camps, 103; pellagra, 169; rickets, 58, 169; scurvy, 16, 48, 58, 103, 169
De humani corporis fabrica libri septem, 68
Dental cavities, 59, 60
Dental lesions, 58–59, 60, 61
Dental tools, 39, *40*
Dentists, 37–40
Diet and food, 168–69, 178–79. See also Vegetarianism
Disease, influence of topography and local conditions, 90–91
Disease and Discrimination (Hutchinson), 189
Disinfectants, 134. See also Infectious disease
Dissection, anatomical, 72, 74, 77–81
Distillation, 25
Doctoresses, 32, 35–36
Doctors. See Physicians
Dogwood *(Cornus florida)*, 16
Doiry, Edward Sr., 169
Domestic health care. See Home health care in colonial era

Domestic Medicine (Buchan), 30–31
Domestic Medicine, or Poor Man's Friend (Gunn), 31
Donahue, Dr., of New Brunswick, New Jersey, 92
Donahue, John (Five Points District brothel owner), 54, 120–21
Drake, Daniel, 65, 89–91
Dr. Barnett's Parlor Gymnasium, 177
Dreams, and disease, 12–13
Dr. Henley's California IXL Bitters, 154
Dr. McClean's Strengthening Cordial and Blood Purifier, 154
Dr. McMunn's Elixir of Opium, 154
Dr. Sweet's Infallible Liniment, 153
Dr. William's Pink Pills for Pale People, 153
Dr. Worden's Female Pills for all Female Diseases, 164
Dust, in domestic settings, 126
Dwarf tapeworms *(Hymenolepiasis nana)*, 121

Earhart, Amelia, 181
Earth closets, 126, *127*
Eastlake Houses, 127
Electricity and therapy, 136, 174–75
The Electric Physician (Britten), 175
Embalming, 110, *111*
Emetics, 15, 21, 152
Emmenagogues, 29–30, 35, 164
English Poor Law (1601), 56
Epilepsy, 21
Ether, 93, 106
European health care traditions: blended with African and Native American traditions, 2, 4–5; on cause of disease, 20–21; faith and healing, 19–20; treatments for disease, 21–22
Ewell, Thomas, 31
Excavation sites. *See* Archaeological sites
Excelsior spring water, 174
Exercise, 175–78

Fairbanks, Douglas, 174
Family cures, 2. *See also* Women's roles in healing

Family life: erosion of, 64; privatization of, 45–46
The Family Physician (Benezet), 31
"Family right certificates," 87–88
Fawcett, Lawrence, 159
F. Brown's Essence of Jamaica Ginger, 154
Feather beds, 128
Febrifuges, 16, 152
Fecal contamination. *See* Hygiene, public
Ferguson, Leland, *18*, 19
Fetoscopes. *See* Stethoscopes
Firestone, Harvey, 181
Fisher, Charles L., 120
Fisk, Almond, 70
Fisk Coffins, 70–71
Fitness (exercise), 175–78
Fit or Fat (Bailey), 181
Five Points District (Manhattan), 52–54, 120–21
Fleming, Alexander, 50
Fletcher, Horace, 169
Fletcherization, 169
Flint blades, 15
Food, Drug, and Cosmetic Act (1938), 163
Food, Drug, and Cosmetic Act amendments (1962), 163
Food and diet, 168–69, 178–79. *See also* Vegetarianism
Ford, Henry, 181
Formento, Felix, 97
Four humours, 20
Fractures, treatment with splints, 14–15
Friendly Botanic Societies, 87–88
Frogs in the stomach, 30
Fuller, Samuel, 14–15
Funeral expenses, 69–71
Funerary trade, 68–73
Funk, Casimir, 169

Galen, 20, 131–32, 170
Gallipots, 25, 155
Galvanic belts, 175, 179
Gangrene, 107
Germ theory, 20, 131–32, 133–34
Gleizmann, Dr. Joseph, 142
Godey's Lady's Book, 127

Goforth, Dr., 89
Goldenseal *(Hydrastis canadensis)*, 16
Goldin, Grace, 99–101
Gove, Mary, 86. *See also* Nichols, Mary Gove
Graham, Dr. James, 38–39
Graham, Sylvester, 86, 88, 168, 178
Grand State Celestial Bed, 38–39
Granula, 180
Grauer, Anne L., 61
Grave robbing, 69–70
"The Great American Medical Fraud" (Adams), 162
Greenwood, Dr. John, 39
Griscom, Dr. John, 124–25
Grob, Gerald N., 45
Guided practice and healing, 178–81
A Guide for Women (Pinkham), 151
Gunn, J. C., 31
Gymnastics, 176
Gynecology, 28–30, 92–94. *See also* Midwives

Hahnemann, Samuel, 88
HAI (healthcare-associated infections), 91, 131
Haines, Michael R., 57–58
Hale, Mary, 36
Hall, Mary Ann, 51–52
Hamlin, John A., 160
Hamlin's Wizard Oil, *153*, 160
Hammond, Dr. William A. (Surgeon General), 99, 101, 103, 105, 108, 109–10, 112
Handbooks: for domestic health care, 30–32; recipe books, 24
Harding, Warren, 181
Harewood Hospital, *102*
Harrington, Judith M., 78
Harris, Elisha, 107
Hayes, Isaac, 101
Healing, phenomenological approaches to, 13
Health care in U.S., current, 1
Health reformers, nineteenth century, 7, 86
Healy, John, 160
Heeregraft (canal), 117–18

Hellebore *(Veratrum viride)*, 15, 16, 152
Hemlock *(Conium maculatum)*, 15, 152
Herbalism and herbal remedies. *See* Plant recipes for healing
Hering, Constantine, 88
Heroic medicine, 83–85
Highland Park Skeletal Collection, 60
Hippocrates, 20
Historic documents, 2
Hitchcock, Edward, 86
Hodge, Hugh Lenox, 92
Holmes' Fragrant Frostilla for the Toilet, 154
Home health care in colonial era: apothecaries, 37–38; care of children, 26–28; care of the sick, 24–26; care of women's conditions, 28–30; clerics, 36–37; dentists, 37–38; doctoresses, 35–36; handbooks, 30–32; home cures, 2, 4; itinerant physicians, 38–40; midwives, 32–35; overview, 183–84; physicians, professionally trained, 37
Homeopathic medicine, 88
Hooker's Division, 51–52
Hookworms *(Necator americanus)*, 119, 122
Hopkins, Anthony, 179
Horlick's Malted Milk, 154, 166
Hospital-acquired infections, 91, 131
Hospitalism, 91, 98, 133
Hospitals: during Civil War, 99–103; field hospitals, 101; general hospitals, 62–64, 101; hospital design, 131, 133; hospital reform, 131–34; pavilion design, 99–101, *100*, 131, 133, 145; for seamen, 48; and sterilization, 133–34
Hostetter's Stomach Bitters, 153, 162
Hotel Hot Sulfur Wells, 173
Hot Wells Hotel/Park, 173
Household Manual of Domestic Hygiene, Food and Diet (Kellogg), 127
How the Other Half Lives (Riis), 52
Human waste disposal. *See* Hygiene, public
Humoural theory of disease, 20, 28–29, 83–85
Hunkin, Tim, 39
Hunter, John, 73
Hunter, William, 73

Huntington, David Low (D. L.), 108, 113
Huron people, 13
Hydropathy and hydrotherapy, 170, *171*
Hygiene, personal, 129
Hygiene, public: fecal contamination and sewage, 116–22; hygiene in the home, 127–29; and public health, 185; rural sanitation, 122; water sources and sanitary reform, 122–27

Immigration, 45–46
Indian Pink *(Spigelia marilandica)*, 15, 16, 24, 152
Indian Removal Act, 82
Indians, American. *See* Native American health care traditions
Indian tobacco *(Lobelia inflata)*, 24, 87
Industrialization, 45–46
Infant mortality, 61
Infectious disease: Civil War wounds, 104, 107–8; hospital acquired, 91, 131; and Native Americans, 11; and urban crowding, 46
Influenza pandemic (1918), 189
Inoculation, 37
Internal balance, 15
Intestinal parasites, 119–20, 121, 152
Ipecac, 85
Iroquois people, 12, 14, 15, 16, 152

Jackson, Andrew, 82, 85, 184
Jackson, James C., 86
Jacksonian movement, 85–87, 90, 161
Jamaican senna *(Cassia obovata)*, 24
Jamestown, Virginia, 115
Jerusalem Oak *(Chenopodium ambrosioides)*, 15, 24, 53
Jimsonweed *(Datura stramonium)*, 53
Joe Pye weed *(Eutrochium purpureum)*, 16
Johns Hopkins Hospital, 133
Johnson, Andrew, 105
Johnson's Island, 112
Jones, Dr. Joseph, 98
Josselyn, John, 16
Journal of the American Medical Association (JAMA), 89

Kelley, James E., *109*
Kellogg, John Harvey, 7, 88, 128, 169, 170, 178–81
Kellogg, William Keith, 180–81
Kellogg Company, 180
Kelly, Elizabeth, 21
Kesey, Ken, 141
Kickapoo Indian Medicine Company, 160
Kickapoo Indian Oil, 163
Kirkbride, Thomas Story, 137
Kirkbride plan, 137
Kitchen medicine and gardens, 25
Klepp, Susan, 30
Koch, Robert, 132, 133–34, 142
Kongo Cosmogram, *18*, 19
Kresge, S. S., 181

Laënnec, Théophile-René-Hyacinthe, 164
Lancets, *84*, 106
Landscapes, physical, and health, 5
Lane, Roger, 55
Lawson, John, 11, 13
Laxatives, 15
Lay health reformers, nineteenth century, 86
Lay practitioners, 32
Leadbeater, John, 157
Learned Quackery Exposed (Thomson), 86–87
LeGear's Screw Worm Killer, 153
Letterman, Jonathan, 103
Lewis, Dioclesian, 176
Licorice *(Glycyrrhiza glabra)*, 24
Lincoln, Mary Todd, 181
Lister, Joseph, 132
Listerine, 132
Lloyd's Cocaine Tooth Drops, 153
Lobelia *(Lobelia inflata)*, 15, 87
Lydia Pinkham's Vegetable Compound, 149–52, *150*, 162, 164

Macfadden, Bernarr, 177–78
Macracanthorhynchus hirudinaceus (zoonotic parasite), 121
Madder *(Rubia tinctorum)*, 29
Madison Springs, 172

Magic, 21
Malaria, 46, 104
Malleus Malleficarum, 21
Malnutrition. *See* Deficiency diseases
A Manual of Free Gymnastic and Dumb-Bell Exercises (Stuart), 176
Maritime trades, 47–49
Massachusetts General Hospital, 48, 136
Mastication (Fletcherization), 169
Maternal mortality, 28
Mather, Cotton, 36–37
Matthews, William, 31
Mattresses, 128–29
Mayapple *(Podophyllum peltatum)*, 15, 16, 152
Mayo, Charles, 179
Mayo, William, 179
Medical and Surgical History of the War of the Rebellion, 108, 112
Medical doctors. *See* Physicians
Medical schools, 66–68, 82–85
Medical societies, 83
Medicine shows, 159–60
Mehta, Jayur, 13–14
Mellin's Infant's Food, 166
Menstruation, 28–29, 30. *See also* Emmenagogues
Mental illness: institutional care, 135–41; moral treatment for, 137–40
Mercury, 50
Mesmer, Franz Anton, 175
Metropolis Water Act (London), 125–26
Miasmatic theory, 20, 133
Middleton, Peter, 66
Midwife's Book (Sharp), 32
Midwives, 17, 26, 32–35, 163–66
Mineral springs, 170–74
Mineral water cures, 171–72
Ministers: minister-physicians, 65; as physical healers, 21–22. *See also* Home health care in colonial era: clerics
Monroe County Poorhouse, 59–60
Moore, Samuel Preston, 104
Moral treatment for mental illness, 137–40
Morgan, J. P., 174
Morphine, 106
Morrogh, Dr. Clifford, 91–93, 106

Mortality: childhood and maternal, 28; infant, 61
Mortsafes, *70*
Moseley folding bathrub, *128*, 129
Munson, Dr. James, 140

National Medical Convention, 88
Native American health care traditions: blended with European and African traditions, 2, 4–5; on cause of disease, 12–13; faith and healing, 12; and infectious disease, 11; medical treatments, 11–12; plant knowledge, 152; treatments for disease, 13–16
Natural Hot Sulphur Wells, 173
Naylor, Katherine, 119–20
Neurasthenia, 172–73
New Family Physician (Gunn), 31
New Gymnastics for Men, Women, and Children (Lewis), 176
New Haven Hospital, 48
New York Abortion Act (1845), 55
New York (New Amsterdam) and public hygiene, 117
New York Hygeio-Therapeutic College, 171
Nichols, Mary Gove, 171. *See also* Gove, Mary
Nichols, Thomas, 171
Nightingale, Florence, 131
Northern Michigan Asylum, 137–41, *138, 139, 141*
Nosocomially acquired infections, 91, 131
Nuttose, 180–181
Nystrom, Kenneth C., 74–75, 76

Oak *(Quercus sp.)*, 15, 152
Obama, Barack, 1
Obstetrics, 163–66. *See also* Midwives
Occupational hazards, 47
O'Followell, Ludovic, 176
Ojibwa people, 15, 16
Okra *(Abelmoschus esculentus)*, 24
One Flew Over the Cuckoo's Nest (Kesey), 141
Opium, 85
Osteomalacia, 58
Otis, George A., 108–9, 110, 112–13
Our Homes (Murphy), 127

Paine's Celery Compound, 153
Parasites, intestinal, 119–20, 121, 152
Paris Clinical School, 73
Parker, Edgar Randolph, 39–40
Parker Dental Circus, 40
Parks, Amanda L., 14
Pasteur, Louis, 132
Patent medicines, 151–54, 166–167; regulation of, 161–63
Pavilion hospital design, 99–101, *100*, 131, 133, 145
Peanut butter, 180–81
Pellagra, 169
Penney, J. C., 181
Pennsylvania Hospital, 135, 136, 137
Pennyroyal *(Hedeoma puegiodes)*, 29
Peoria City Cemetery, 60–61
Peoria Sanatorium, 145
Perryman, Lucrecia, 165–66
Personal hygiene, 129
Pessaries, 92
Pest houses, 46
Pharmacy schools, 154–55; and equipment, 155–56
Phlegm, humoural theory, 20
Physical culture, 176
Physical Culture (periodical, Bernarr Macfadden editor), 177–78
Physicians: contrasted with apothecaries, 155, 161–62; contrasted with midwives, 163–66; criticism of, 88–91; income of, 89–90; licensure of, 89; public distrust of, 83, 85–88, 184; social status of, 65–66; training of, 37, 65, 88–89; women as, 104–5
Physiology and Calisthenics (Beecher), 176
Pill rollers, *156*
Pima people, 15
Pinkham, Lydia Estes, 149
Pinkroot *(Spigelia marilandica)*, 15, 16, 152
Pitch doctors at medicine shows, 159–60
Plant recipes for healing: African, 17–19; during colonial era, 24–25; herbal remedies, 87–88, 152; Native American, 15–16; preservation of plants, 25; used in brothels, 53. *See also specific plant names*
Plath, Sylvia, 141

Plum, wild *(Prunus americana)*, 15
Pond's Extract, 154
Poorhouses, 50, 55–61, 74–77
Population density, early U.S., 16, 45–46
Post, C. W., 181
Poverty, 6, 46–47, 55–56, 185
Powhatan people, 13, 15
A Practical Treatise on the Medical and Surgical Uses of Electricity, 175
Pregnancy, 26, 29, 54–55. *See also* Midwives
Primitive Physick (Wesley), 31–32
Principles of Domestic Science (Beecher and Stowe), 127
Prisoners of war, 110–12
Privatization of family life, 45–46
Privies, use of and archaeological value of, 116–20
Privy laws, 118
Prosthetic limbs, *109*
Prostitution, 50–55, 120–21
Psychiatric facilities. *See* Asylums for special needs patients
Public hygiene. *See* Hygiene, public
Puke weed *(Lobelia inflata)*, 87
Pure Food and Drug Act (1906), 151, 152, 163

Quackery, 30–31, 162
Queen Anne's Revenge (QAR), 48–49

Raccoon *(Procyon lotor)*, 16
Recipe books for treatments, 24
Reciprocity, 12
Red cedar *(Juniperus virginiana L.)*, 29
Redeemer community, 14
Reed, Walter, 113
Reid, David Boswell, 123
Reinhard, Karl, 53, 121
Restraints, physical, in asylums, 135–36, *136*
Resurrection men, 69–70
Revisionist movements in medicine, 85–88
Rickets, 58, 169
Ridge ventilation, 99, 133
Riis, Jacob, 52
Risky trades, 47
The Road to Wellville (Boyle), 179
Robson, Dr., 120
Rochdale Pail System, 122

Rockefeller, John D., 122
Rockefeller Sanitary Commission, 122
Röentgen, Wilhelm Conrad, 176
Rogers, Will, 174
Roger's Cocaine Pile Remedy, 153
Roosevelt, Teddy, 174
Root beer, 152
Rosenberg, Charles, 130
Roundworms *(Ascaris lumbricoides)*, 119, 121
Ruble, Thomas W., 31
Rural sanitation, 122
Rush, Benjamin, 83, 135

Sailors, 47–49
Salem witch trials, 21
The Sanitary Condition of the Laboring Population (Griscom), 124–25
Sanitation. *See* Hygiene, public
Sappol, Michael, 65, 72
Saranac Lake sanatorium, 142–44, *143*
Saratoga Springs, 172
Sassafras *(Sassafras albidum)*, 16, 30, 152
Satterlee Hospital, 101, *102*
Savin *(Juniperus sabina L.)*, 29
Saw palmetto *(Serenoa repens)*, 19
Scarificators, *84*
Schultz, Jane, 104–5
Science-based medicine, criticism of, 88–91
Scurvy, 16, 48, 58, 103, 169
Semisubterranean sweat lodges (SSLs), 14
Seneca Snakeroot *(Polygala senega)*, 15–16, 29
Seriation (archaeological dating technique), 3–4
Seventh-day Adventists, 168–69, 178
Sewage. *See* Hygiene, public
Sexually transmitted diseases, 185
Sex work, 50–55, 120–21
Shamans, 12
Sharp, Dr. (medical specialist from London), 38
Sharp, Jane, 23, 32
Shew, Joel, 171
Shippen, William, 163
Sick-building syndrome, 185
Sierra Leone, and Colonoware, 19
Simpson, Dr. James, 93

Sims, James Marion, 92, 94
Skeletal lesions, 58, 60, 61
Skeletal remains, 54–55, 58, 60, 76–81; and ancestry estimates, 77
Slave communities, 17–18
Sleeping porches, 143–44
Sleeping quarters, 128–29
Smallpox, 36–37
Smith, Dr. William Lay, 89
Smith, John, 115
Smith, Michael, 36
Snow, Dr. John, 125
Social stratification, 5–6, 85, 184–85
Sources: archaeological, 3–4; documents, 2
Spanish fly, 84–85
Spas, 172–74
Spirituality: and health, 86; spiritual basis of disease, 21–22
Splints, to treat fractures, 14–15
Spruce *(Picea* sp.), 16
Stabler, Edward, 156–57
Stabler, William, 157
Stabler-Leadbeater shop, 156–59, *157, 158*
Standing stools, 27
Stanton, Edwin M., 103, 109
Sterilization in hospitals, 133–34
Stethoscopes, 164
Stills, metallic, 25
Stout, Samuel, 104
Strachey, William, 115
Supplements, vitamin, 169
Surgery, 63–64; surgeons, 65; surgical equipment, *108. See also* Amputation
Surinam Poison, 24
Swaddling of infants, 27
Sweat lodges, 13–14
Syphilis, 50, 185
Syringes: urethral, *49*; vaginal, 92
Szent-Györgyi, Albert, 169

Tannins, 15
Tapeworms *(Taenia saginata)*, 119, 121
Tartar emetic (antimony), 108, 110
Taylor, Dr. Augustus F., 93
Thatch, Edward, 48
Thompson, Dr. Frank, 80
Thompson, John D., 99–101

Thomson, Samuel, 86–88, 149
Thomsonians, 86, 149
Thucydides, 131–32
Tobacco (*Nicotiana* sp.), 16
Trail of Tears, 87
Trall, Russell, 171
Tranquilizer chair, *136*
Traverse City State Hospital, 137–41, *138*, *139*, *141*
Treatise of Domestic Medicine (Cooper), 31
Treatise on Domestic Medicine (Matthews), 31
Trommer's Extract of Malt, 154
Trudeau, Dr. Edward Livingston, 142–43
Trudeau Institute, 144
Trump, Donald, 187–88
Tuberculosis (TB), 128, 142
Tuberculosis sanatoria, 142–45
Turpentine, 30
Tyndall, John, 134

United States Sanitary Commission, 123
Universe, cyclical nature of, 12
Urbanization, 45–46, 64
Urethral syringes, *49*
The Uses of Water in Health and Disease (Kellogg), 170
U.S. Pharmacopoeia, 15
Uxbridge Almshouse, 69

Vaginal syringes, 92
Valentino, Rudolph, 174
Vegetarianism, 88, 168–169
Vegetine the Great Blood Purifier, 153
Ventilation, 123, 128, 131, 133, 137, 139; ridge ventilation, 99, 133
Ventilation in Americn Dwellings (Reid), 123
Vermifuges, 15, 152
Vesalius, 68
Vitamin C, 16, 58. *See also* Scurvy
Vitamin supplements, 169

Wage labor, 45–46
Walker, Mary Edwards, 105
Walker, Philip, 58
Walking stools, 27–28
Ward, Montgomery, 181

Warner's Safe Cure, 153
Washington, George, 39, 85
Water closets, 123–24
The Water-Cure Journal, 170, 171
Water supplies. *See* Hygiene, public
Water therapy, 170–74
Waverly Hills, 145
Weissmuller, Johnny, 181
Welch, Edgar, 181
Wells, public, 117
Wells, W. R., 175
Wesley, John, 31–32
Western Health Reform Institute, 178
Western Resorts for Health and Pleasure . . ., 173
Whaling, 48
Whipworms *(Trichuris trichiura)*, 121
White, Ellen G., 178, 179
White willow *(Salix alba)*, 16
Wild cherry *(Prunus avium)*, 15
Wild geranium *(Geranium maculatum)*, 15, 152
Wild plum *(Prunus americana)*, 15
Wilkie, Laurie A., 166
William Radam's Microbe Killer, 153
Williamsburg, VA, Public Hospital, 136
Witchcraft, 21, 36
Women's rights and fitness programs, 176
Women's roles in healing, 24. *See also* Doctoresses; Home health care in colonial era; Midwives
Wood, Alexander, 106
Woodward, Joseph J., 113
Workhouses, 50, 55–61, 74–77
Workplace hazards, 47
Wormseed *(Chenopodium ambrosioides)*, 15, 53
Wounds, battlefield, 105, 107
Wyatt, Sir Francis, 115

X-rays, 176

Yaupon *(Ilex vomitoria)*, 15
Yellow bile, in humoural theory, 20
Yellow fever, 46, 113
Young, James Harvey, 161

DALE L. HUTCHINSON is professor emeritus of anthropology at the University of North Carolina (UNC) at Chapel Hill; his teaching and research are focused on the health and nutrition of present and past populations, disease ecology, forensic anthropology, and mortuary archaeology. He is also affiliated at the same institution with the Research Laboratories of Archaeology and the Institute of Arts and Humanities. Beyond UNC, he is a Fellow of the American Association for the Advancement of Science.